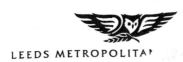
LEEDS METROPOLITAN

HEALTH & COMMUNITY

HEALTH &
COMMUNITY

Holism in Practice

EDITED BY MIKE MONEY

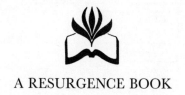

A RESURGENCE BOOK

A Resurgence Book
First published in 1993 by
Green Books Ltd
Foxhole, Dartington,
Totnes, Devon TQ9 6EB, UK

© Green Books Ltd
The individual chapters are the copyright of the authors.

Designed by David Baker

Typeset by Ian D. Luckett,
St. Austell, Cornwall

Printed by Biddles Ltd
Guildford, Surrey

A catalogue record for this book is available from
the British Library

ISBN 1 870098 53 6 ✓

Contents

Introduction

This is a book about health, and it has as its focus the relationship between health and community. There are a number of reasons for producing it, and it may be helpful to the reader to know what they are.

First, the book preserves in a more permanent form some excellent articles which have appeared in *Resurgence* magazine over the last fifteen years. These articles are written by a range of people and from a variety of contexts, but they all focus upon notions of health and the ways in which health is a community matter. I have introduced each article with a brief account of its relevance to the theme of community and health, and incorporated references to guide the interested reader to further material. In some cases these references have been recently provided by the author of the article; in many cases they are my own suggestions.

There are many ways of thinking about health, and none of them is exclusively right or definitively wrong. You can think of health as freedom from pain or disease, and when you are ill or in pain this can seem a very good way to think of it. But while a General Practitioner can do a lot if you've caught something nasty, there's no vaccination against being knocked down by a car, and no drug to cure bad housing. Over the last fifty years people have explored the idea that there is more to health than medical intervention, that health can be thought of as a positive state, in the same sense that warmth isn't just absence of cold but a more positive sensation altogether.

But the question arises, how do we move into this more positive state of health? On the whole, people have given three sorts of answers, and all of them have some validity. There are those who say you must focus on the individual, because in the end all change begins when a person chooses to do something different. Some focus on the national or international level of action, arguing that only with changes in govern-mental policy or international law will the real issues — such as pollution, poverty or famine — be addressed.

But this book focuses on the community. It does so not only because in recent years this has been the tendency of some health-related bodies — such as the World Health Organization — but also because of my own involvement in health and community, which goes back about twenty years. Like many other people, I have become convinced that you can only be a healthy person if you are a part of a healthy community. I think this is true for a wide range of issues that includes mental health (and I don't just mean the care of mental illness, though it's true there too), air and water quality, nutrition, and physical safety. For many health issues, the isolated individual is powerless and national government may be indifferent or even hostile. This is where communities come in, and one of the assumptions on which this book is based is that local communities are the experts on themselves, their own needs, and how those needs should be met.

The book is addressed to at least three sorts of people. It is for those already at work in community action of some sort, and who I hope will find in it ideas that inspire them to continue and expand their work. It is for students in any discipline which has relevance to health — and these days there are few disciplines which do not — in the hope that they will find the articles inspirational and the further reading instructive. And thirdly it is for those who like myself have the privilege of teaching such students and who I hope will find, as I did, that the materials here give an essential practical focus to the subject of community health and community development.

Mike Money
Hooton, Cheshire
June 1993

PART ONE

BELONGING
TO THE LAND

Introduction to Gary Snyder

RE-INHABITATION

When planning this book, I gave a lot of thought to the sequence of the articles. But whichever way around I experimented, Gary Snyder's piece always came first. So it introduces both the book as a whole and specifically the section *Belonging to the Land*.

This is because Snyder's contribution is fundamental to concepts of healthy community, reminding us that at the heart of notions of physical and mental health is the notion of belonging. We are herd animals, we are tribal animals (or ought to be) and we are territorial animals. We may not be territorial in the ways of some species, we may not need to mark out a new territory each season, but we do need to identify with some particular spot on the planet's surface. Just as we need to identify and find ourselves in the context of family and friends, so we need to know the physical place where we belong. We cherish our place and it nurtures us.

Ultimately, all lives and all health — however defined — rest quite literally upon the earth; and unless we remain or become what Snyder calls 'inhabitants' we will never come to the grounded view that earth is sacred. We will be perpetual transients; treating each temporary resting-place as something to be consumed, excreted and abandoned — a practice which will ultimately consume the planet. The alternative is to see our spot as somewhere sacred, to which we belong as much as it belongs to us, in which the generations of the past share as equals, and in which all species and elements have an equitable stake.

The discipline of health promotion is beginning to recognise the vital nature of an ecological perspective — that however hard the individual strives for health, health is impossible if the planet is poisoned. Snyder articulates the philosophical premises of this position: a healthy community is impossible if the physical conditions for good health are denied. It requires the cooperative action of the community for a healthy environment to be recovered, maintained and enhanced. Only community action can safeguard the physical base in which that community is rooted.

The WHO Ottawa Charter spoke of advocacy, mediation and enablement. One aspect of mediation is to speak for the land; to be its advocate. The realisation of this process can be empowering; for there are many instances of community definition and development that have grown out of the perception of a threat to the community place — dam building, motorway construction, air pollution. Snyder's article demonstrates the importance for mental and physical community health of us all becoming reinhabitants of the places where we live.

FURTHER READING

Daniel Chodorkoff (1990) **Social Ecology and Community Development** in J. Clark (Ed) *Renewing the Earth*. Green Print, pp 60–70.

Mike Money (1992) **Health education, Ecology, and the Shamanic World View** *Health Education Research* Vol 7 Part 2, pp 301-303.

John Seed et al (1988) **Thinking Like a Mountain**. New Society Publications.

Gary Snyder (1990) **Regenerate Culture!** in *Turtle Talk — Voices for a sustainable future* Christopher and Judith Plant (Eds). New Society Pubs., pp 12–22.

World Health Organisation (1992) **Our planet, our health**. WHO.

RE-INHABITATION

GARY SNYDER

I CAME HERE BY A PATH, a line, of people that somehow worked their way from the Atlantic seaboard westward over 150 years. One grandfather ended up in the Territory of Washington, and homesteaded in Kitsap County. My mother's side was railroad people down in Texas, and before that they'd worked the silver mines in Leadville, Colorado. My grandfather, being a homesteader, and my father a native of the state of Washington, put our family relatively early in the North-west. Yet we weren't early enough. An elderly Salish Indian gentleman came by our farm once every few months in a model T truck, selling smoked salmon. "Who is he?" "He's an Indian" my parents said —

Looking at all the different trees and plants that made up my second-growth Douglas fir forest plus cow-pasture childhood universe, I realized that my parents were short on a certain kind of knowledge. They could say "That's a Doug fir, that's a cedar, that's bracken fern…" But I perceived a subtlety and complexity in those woods that went far beyond a few names.

As a child I spoke with the old Salishan man a few times over the years he made these stops — then, suddenly, he never came back. I sensed what he represented, what he knew, and what it meant to me: he knew better than anyone else I had ever met, *where I was*. I had no notion of a white American or European heritage providing an identity; I defined myself by relation to the place. Soon I also understood that "English language" is an identity — and later, via the hearsay of books, received the full cultural and historical view — but never forgot, or left, that first ground: the "where" of our "who are we?"

There are many people on the planet, now, who are not "inhabit-ants". Far from their home villages; removed from ancestral territories; moved into town from the farm; went to pan gold in California — work on the Pipeline — work for Bechtel in Iran. Actual inhabitants — peasants, paisanos, paysan, peoples of the land, have been sniffed at,

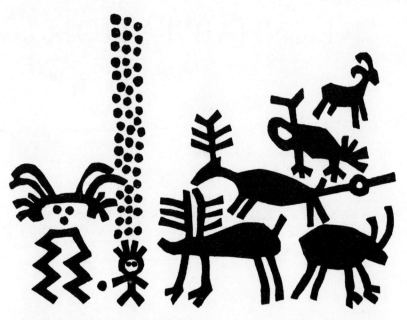

laughed at, and overtaxed for centuries by the urban-based ruling elites. The intellectuals haven't the least notion of what kind of sophisticated, attentive, creative intelligence it takes to "grow food". Virtually al the plants in the gardens and the trees in the orchards, the sheep, cows and goats in the pastures were domesticated in the Neolithic; before "civilization". The differing regions of the world have long had — each — their own precise subsistence pattern developed over millennia by people who had settled in there and learned what particular kinds of plant the ground would "say" at that spot.

Humankind also clearly wanders. Four million years ago those smaller proto-humans were moving in and out of the edges of forest and grassland in Africa; fairly warm; open enough to run in. At some point moving on, catching fire, sewing clothes, swinging around the arctic, setting out on amazing sea voyages. A skull found in Santa Barbara has been dated at 50,000 years. So it may be that during the middle and late Pleistocene, large fauna hunting era, a fairly nomadic grassland-and-tundra hunting life was established, with lots of mobility across northern Eurasia in particular. With the decline of the Ice Age — and here's where we are, most of the big game hunters went out of business. There was possibly a population drop in Eurasia and the Americas, as the old techniques no longer worked.

Countless local ecosystem habitation styles emerged. People developed specific ways to be in each of those niches: plant knowledge, boats, dogs, traps, nets, fishing — the smaller animals, and smaller tools. From steep jungle slopes of Southwest China to coral atolls to barren arctic deserts — *a spirit of what it was to be there evolved*, that spoke of a direct sense of relation to the "land" — which really means, the totality of the local bio-region system, from cirrus clouds to leaf-mould.

So, inhabitory peoples sometimes say "this piece of land is sacred" — or "all the land is sacred." This is an attitude that draws on awareness of the mystery of life and death; of taking life to live; of giving life back — not only to your own children, but to the life of the whole land.

Abbé Breuil, the French prehistorian who worked extensively in the caves of southern France, has pointed out that the animal murals in those 20,000-year-old caves describe fertility as well as hunting — the birth of little bison and cow calves. They show a tender and accurate observation of the qualities and personalities of different creatures; implying a sense of the mutuality of life and death in the food chain; and what I take to be a sense of a sacramental quality in that relationship.

Inhabitation does not mean "not travelling". The term does not of itself define the size of a territory. The size is determined by the bio-region type. The bison hunters of the great plains are as surely in a "territory" as the Indians of northern California, though the latter may have seldom ventured farther than thirty miles from where they were born. Whether a vast grassland, or a brushy mountain, the Peoples knew their geography. Any member of a hunting society could project from his visualization any spot in the surrounding landscape, and tell you what was there; how to get there. "That's where you'd get some cat-tails." The bushmen of the Kalahari desert could locate a buried ostrich egg full of emergency water in the midst of a sandy waste — walk right up and dig it out, "I put this here three years ago, just in case."

Ray Dasmann has useful terms to make these distinctions: "ecosystem-based cultures" and "biosphere cultures". By that Ray means societies whose life and economies are centred in terms of natural regions and watersheds, as against those who discovered — 7,000 or 8,000 years ago in a few corners of the globe — that it was "profitable" to spill over into another drainage, another watershed, another people's territory, and steal away its resources, natural or human. Thus the

Roman Empire would strip whole provinces for the benefit of the capital, and villa-owning Roman aristocrats would have huge slave-operated farms in the south using giant wheeled ploughs. Southern Italy never recovered. We know the term "imperialism" — Dasmann's "biosphere cultures" adds to that, helps us realize that biological exploitation is a critical part of it too — the species made extinct. The clear-cut forests.

All that wealth and power pouring into a few centres had bizarre results. Philosophies and religions based on fascination with society, hierarchy, manipulation, and the "absolute". A great edifice called "the state" and the symbols of central power — in China what they used to call "the true dragon"; in the West, as Mumford says, symbolized perhaps by that bronze age fort called the Pentagon. No wonder Lévi-Strauss says that civilization has been in a long decline since the Neolithic.

So here in the twentieth century we find occidentals and orientals studying each other's Wisdom, and a few people on both sides studying what came before both — before they forked off. A book like *Black Elk Speaks*, which would probably have had zero readership in 1900, is perceived now as speaking of certain things that nothing in the Judaeo-Christian tradition, and almost nothing in the Hindu-Buddhist tradition, deals with. All the great civilized world religions remain primarily human-centred. That next step is excluded, or forgotten — "Well, what do you say to Magpie? What do you say to Rattlesnake when you meet him?" What do we learn from Wren, and Hummingbird, and Pine Pollen, and how? Learn what? Specifics: how to spend a life facing the current; or what it is to perpetually die young; or how to be huge and calm and eat *anything* (Bear). But also, that we are many selves looking at each other, through the same eye.

The reason many of us want to make this step is simple, and is explained in terms of the 40,000 year looping back that we seem to be involved in. Sometime in the last ten years the best brains of the Occident discovered to their amazement that we live in an Environment. This discovery has been forced on us by the realization that we are approaching the limits of something. Stewart Brand said that the photograph of the earth (taken from outer space by a satellite) that shows the whole blue orb with spirals and whorls of cloud, was a great landmark for human consciousness. We see that it has a shape, and it has limits. We are back again, now, in the position of our Mesolithic forebears — working off the coasts of southern Britain, or the shores of

Lake Chad or the swamps of south-east China, learning how to live by the sun and the green at that spot. We once more know that we live in a system that is enclosed in a certain way; that has its own kinds of limits, and that we are interdependent with it.

THE ETHICS OR MORALITY of this is far more subtle than merely being nice to squirrels. The biological-ecological sciences have been laying out (implicitly) a spiritual dimension. We must find our way to seeing the mineral cycles, the water cycles, air cycles, nutrient cycles, as sacramental — and we must incorporate that insight into our own personal spiritual quest and integrate it with all the wisdom teachings we have received from the nearer past. The expression of it is simple; gratitude to it all, taking responsibility for your own acts; keeping contact with the sources of the energy that flow into your own life (i.e. dirt, water, flesh).

Another question is raised: Is not the purpose of all this living and studying the achievement of self-knowledge, self-realization? How does knowledge of place help us know the Self? The answer, simply put, is that we are all composite beings, not only physically but intellectually, whose sole individual identifying feature is a particular form or structure changing constantly in time. There is no "self" to be found in that, and yet oddly enough, there is. Part of you is out there waiting to come into you, and another part of you is behind you, and the "just this" of the ever-present moment holds all the transitory little selves in its mirror. The Avatamsaka ("Flower Wreath") jewelled-net-interpenetration-eco-logical-systems-emptiness-consciousness tells us, no self-realization without the Whole Self, and the whole self is the whole thing.

Thus, knowing who and where are intimately linked. There are no limits to the possibilities of the study of *who* and *where*, if you want to go "beyond limits" — and so, even in a world of biological limits, there is plenty of open mind-space to go out into.

SUMMING UP, in Wendell Berry's essay "the unsettling of America" he points out that the way the economic system works now, you're penalized if you try to stay in one spot and do anything well. It's not just that the integrity of Native American land is threatened, or National Forests and Parks; it's *all* land that's under the gun, and any person or group of people who tries to stay there and do some one thing well, long enough, to be able to say, "I really love and know this place," stands to be penalized. The economics of it works so that anyone who jumps at the chance for quick profit is rewarded — doing proper agriculture means *not* to jump at the most profitable chance — proper forest management or game management means doing things with the far future in mind — and the future is unable to pay us for it right now. Doing things right means living as though your grandchildren would also be alive, in this land, carrying on the work we're doing right now, with deepening delight.

I saw old farmers in Kentucky last spring who belong in another century. They are inhabitants; they see the world they know crumbling and evaporating before them in the face of a different logic that declares, "everything you know, and do, and the way you do it, means nothing to us." How much more the pain, and loss of elegant cultural skills, on the part of non-white fourth-world primitive remnant cultures — who may know the special properties of a certain plant, or how to communicate with dolphins, skills the industrial world might never regain. Not that special, intriguing knowledges are the real point: it's the sense of the magic system; the capacity to hear the song of Gaia *at that spot*, that's lost.

Re-inhabitory refers to the tiny number of persons who come out of the industrial societies (having collected or squandered the fruits of 8,000 years of civilization) and then start to turn back to the land, to place. This comes for some with the rational and scientific realization of inter-connectedness, and planetary limits. But the actual demands of a life committed to a place, and living somewhat by the sunshine green plant energy that is concentrating in that spot, are so physically and intellectually intense, that it is a moral and spiritual choice as well.

"Mankind has a rendezvous with destiny in Outer Space." Some say. We are already travelling in space. This is the galaxy, right here. The wisdom and skill of those who studied the universe first hand, by direct knowledge and experience, for millennia, both inside and outside themselves, are what we might call the Old Ways. Those who envision a possible future planet on which we continue that study, and where we live by the Green and the Sun, have no choice but to bring whatever science, imagination, strength, and political finesse they have to the support of the inhabitory people — natives and peasants of the world. Entering such paths, we begin to learn a little of the Old Ways, which are outside of history, and forever new.

Gary Snyder is an American author and poet who has been influential in ecological thinking for the last twenty-five years.

This article originally appeared in *The Old Ways*, San Francisco City Lights in 1977. Published under the title 'Earth is Sacred' in *Resurgence* No. 95, November/December 1982.

Introduction to William Greider

THE LAKOTA WANT THE BLACK HILLS BACK

Gary Snyder's article illustrates the importance of reinhabitation; of the need to identify with a land and place of one's own. Greider takes us from principles to practice, demonstrating in detail some of the pragmatic links between community and health. If a community is dispossessed of its land, the consequences for the health of its members are direct and tangible. Conversely, fighting to retain or regain one's place is to find a focus for community regeneration.

This article focuses on one group of dispossessed people, the Lakota. In it Greider explains the nature of the problems they are experiencing — not just dispossession, but the problems that have arisen in its wake. These include extreme poverty, drug addiction, and internal dissent. In 1876, after the Battle of Little Big Horn, the Lakota were forced to leave their Black Hills and settle on reservations. Six years later they were forbidden to practice their religion or speak their own language.

But they have never lost faith that one day they will recover their land. This account shows not only what people have been prepared to endure to retain their links with their land and maintain their identity, but also the importance of the spiritual element in their struggle. The meaning of the struggle impels them to maintain it.

The Lakota are an extreme example of dispossession, but here and now in the United Kingdom and in Europe there are people who are being dispossessed. In some cases that dispossession is literal and physical — people are moved from their homes and communities are dissipated because of a decision to rehouse them in a number of separate areas rather than renovate their existing homes. Sometimes the dispossession seems not so extreme — a motorway divides a community, a planning decision results in blight, or a new runway is built and the community finds it is under a new flightpath. Or new supermarkets and leisure parks take away the vitality of the community.

But the consequences are the same — the community ceases to act as one, social relationships become fragmented, cooperative action ceases. And the implications for physical and mental health are severe. Just as the Lakota have tried to fight back, so many of our own threatened communities are fighting similar battles against an indifferent government. Sometimes the fight is to prevent 'development' that will destroy the community, sometimes to prevent the destruction of some essential community feature such as a school, a library, a wood or meadow. And communities are right to fight such campaigns, because there can be no healthy individuals without healthy communities. At present the sad truth is that many communities are under attack — they have to use their energy for survival rather than enhancement.

The Lakota have persisted in the battle for their 1.3 million acres of land in the Black Hills for over a century, and have refused all offers of financial compensation. The lawsuit for the return of their land was filed in 1923 and is still running. Just as the Lakota have drawn inspiration from the Jews, so other communities — perhaps facing fewer problems — can draw inspiration from the Lakota.

FURTHER READING

Meg Beresford (1988) **We Are All Connected** in Felix Dodds (Ed) *Into The 21st Century*. Green Print, pp 53–67.

Tom Brown Jr & Michael Tobias (1985) **Ancestors** in Michael Tobias (Ed) *Deep Ecology*. Avant Books, pp 122–139.

Angela King & Sue Clifford (1985) **Holding Your Ground** Revised Ed. Wildwood House.

John C. Mowhawk (1990) **Distinguished Traditions** in John Clark (Ed) *Renewing the Earth*. Green Print, pp 91–96.

THE LAKOTA WANT THE
BLACK HILLS BACK

WILLIAM GREIDER

O UTSIDERS KNOW THEM as the Sioux, but they call themselves the Lakota — "the Allies". They once claimed as their own more than 48 million acres in what is now the Dakotas, Nebraska, Wyoming and Montana, lands "set apart" by the United States government in the 1868 Treaty of Fort Laramie "for the absolute and undisturbed use and occupation of the Sioux." That treaty was violated six years later when an expedition led by Lieutenant Colonel George Armstrong Custer discovered gold in the Lakota's sacred Black Hills. After the massacre of Custer and his troops at Little Big Horn in 1876, Congress forced the Lakota to relinquish the Black Hills and to settle on reservations by threatening to cut off their food rations — a choice the Lakota remember as "sell or starve".

The Lakota were not just defeated in battle and deprived of their lands. They were broken as a people. In 1882, the federal Indian agency banned their religion because Indian agents and army officers recognized it as a source of continuing resistance to white occupation; the government prohibited the sun dance, the vision quest and the seven sacred ceremonies. The children of the Lakota attended government schools where they were forbidden to speak their own language.

The Lakota have been a defeated people ever since. Today their poverty is visible on a country road as a Lakota family passes by, its old Comet station wagon chugging along uncertainly. Or in the rickety frame houses of a remote settlement. One cold night on the Pine Ridge reservation I rode alongside a young man as he delivered a load of firewood to an elderly woman whose woodpile was exhausted. She lived in a sagging cabin, hardly bigger than a boxcar, without electricity or plumbing. It was heated by a wood stove, lit by a coal-oil lantern. Pine Ridge is in fact the poorest corner of America, the per capita income of the county the lowest in the nation.

When I first visited Pine Ridge as a young reporter more than fifteen years ago, I experienced the culture shock of visiting a third-world country — only this poverty was right here in America. I was stunned by the harshness of life on the reservation, by the despair in the faces of the young people in the village streets. Some were beautiful faces, recalling the picture-book Indians that children study in school; others were pocked and bloated, with the vacant eyes of young addicts. And as I came to understand more about the Sioux on later visits, the more skeptical I became that any government solution could erase their problems. It was not only the economic barrenness of the reservation or the imperious bureaucracy governing their affairs that crippled the Lakota, for they were a divided people, trapped in bitter arguments, uncertain of their own future.

The Pine Ridge reservation was like a welfare state. Nearly everyone was dependent on the government and the ambitious quarrelled over the scraps of poverty politics. Full bloods resented mixed bloods. "Assimilationists", trying to adapt to white culture, were stubbornly resisted by "traditionalists" who clung to old ways. The 80,000 Lakota still living on or near the reservations were pitted against each other by history. The more I understood these complicated arguments, the more dismal the future seemed to me.

I THINK NOW that I was wrong. Something was stirring among the Lakota even then — a vague but powerful sense of their own heritage. Some young people were taking up old ways and talking to elderly shamans about old secrets. Children were encouraged to study Lakota and to learn the rituals once outlawed. At the time, this cultural revival struck me as a pleasing development but hardly significant alongside the grave conditions on the reservations. When I returned to Pine Ridge after many years, though, I sensed an exciting difference. All of the old arguments continue, the bitter quarrels endure. Yet the Lakota seem to have begun to find a fragile basis for unity, a way to rise above the old arguments of history.

At the heart of this nascent struggle for unity are the Black Hills — the sacred ground the Lakota lost 10 years ago, the core of their spiritual inheritance. After decades of litigation the federal government finally agreed in 1980 to make restitution to the Lakota for the vast lands confiscated from them a century ago. The United States at that time awarded them nearly $105 million for the Black Hills of South Dakota and offered another $39 million for the surrounding lands in other states. But these Indians have done something astounding. In the money-mad eighties, they have refused white America's conscience money. Nearly $200 million — counting interest — sit uncollected in Washington D.C. For some Lakota families, cashing in would mean thousands of dollars. But even the poorest people on the reservations won't touch it. The Lakota want the Black Hills back.

"WE ARE LIKE THE JEWS," Patrick Janis says defiantly. "The Jews always had it in their minds to come back to Israel, and for 2,000 years it was impossible, but they did it. The same with us. Some day we're going to do it. We're going to get back the Black Hills if the people really want it in their hearts.

Janis, 29, tall and square-shouldered, his coarse, wavy hair braided tightly, is himself a fair example of the spiritual revival among the Lakota. Like many Indians, he is of mixed blood — his great-grandfather was one of the white men who served the Sioux chiefs as interpreters, married Indian women and raised their children as Lakota. Four generations later Patrick Janis grew up at Pine Ridge, an angry and alcoholic teenager.

"I was drinking bad, getting in trouble, taking drugs, driving around shooting at people — trying to prove I was a man," he says. Like young Indians on reservations everywhere, Janis saw another America on television and recognized there was no place for him in it. Anything "Indian" was an embarrassment, especially those elders who still mumbled that stuff about spirits and animal brothers and the sacred earth.

"Finally, I decided to quit drinking," Janis says. "I met a guy who was a medicine man, who told me things. He let me sweat with him in the sweat lodge, and I liked it. I started learning how to pray." At twenty-two, after much doubt and meditation, Patrick Janis undertook a once-forbidden ritual, the vision quest known as *hambleceya*. For four days and four nights, he fasted alone on a wilderness peak, seeking guidance from the spirits. "I got a vision up there," he says "which I can't tell you — it's personal and sacred — but it was a vision against alcoholism. It told me to fight against it and protect the children. After I got okay with the spirits, they gave me a medicine man to work with, and I started helping others to sweat. It was good, made them feel good to pray and get clean, but afterward a lot of them started drinking again."

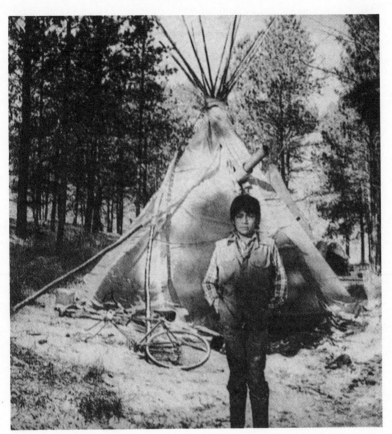

Photo by William Coupon

LIKE MANY OF the young people today, Janis cannot speak Lakota, except for a few words and phrases. He studies old texts left by long-dead holy men, like Blue Horse and Good Seat, which were written down in English by white men. Janis does not pretend that his prayers and rituals are perfect replicas of theirs, but he knows he is speaking with the same spirits.

"I'm still being tested," he says. "The spirits told me, 'Practise humility. Don't hurt anyone around you. Learn how to pray.' I'm still in the process of learning how to pray."

Over the last generation, Lakota ritual and belief has regained vitality, expressed in the communal sun dances held every summer and in individual quests like Janis's. Most of the Lakota have probably not undergone such an awakening. Their gods are still money and booze, as Janis says, and they do not understand all this talk about the sacred Black Hills.

But even the weak and ignorant respond to the issue. Perhaps they recall fragments of what their grandmothers told them as children. Or spooky prophecies they heard from the medicine man around the village. For generations, the Lakota have told their young that if the day ever comes when they sell the Black Hills, all life on earth will perish.

Gerald Clifford — the co-ordinator of the Black Hills steering committee, which was organized by the eight tribal councils as part of the effort to regain ownership of the hills — has witnessed the same eerie moment in dozens of meetings among the Lakota. "When the question of taking the money comes up," Clifford says, "sometimes the talk gets hot and heavy, and people argue. But there's always a moment in these meetings, sooner or later, when someone gets up and gives what might be called the Sacred Earth Speech. What they say, one way or the other, is this 'The Black Hills are our mother. We cannot sell our mother.' There's always an uncanny silence that follows. No one can speak against that. The debate is over."

We cannot sell our mother, even for $200 million.

IN 1976, WHEN the treaty commissioners were imploring Chief Red Cloud to sign away the Black Hills, a warrior named Little Big Man rode into the encampment "singing of bad things to come," as one witness later testified, "He shouted, but they held him back, then he said, 'I will kill any among you that will sell the Black Hills.'"

In 1889, an Oglala leader named Iron Hawk declared to a delegation from Washington, "The Great Spirit has made me and put me on this land, and when he put me here, he made a heart for me, and that is the Black Hills... This land is the Great Spirit's wife, and I am born from there and my heart comes from there. I am Lakota, and I am standing on my own land... We will not sell the land."

In 1918, Eli He Dog, an elderly Sioux chief, made a notarized statement at Pine Ridge, detailing how most chiefs had refused to sell the Black Hills and recounting the long struggle to reclaim them. "I don't know that this will do me any good to make this statement," He Dog testified, "but it may do my children or grandchildren some good. I have been working on this Black Hills claim now for twenty-five years... When I first started this matter, I went all over the reservation, and over $1,150 was collected and counted at Manderson to pay expenses of delegates to go to Washington."

In 1980, a group of Lakota elders — among them Charles Wisespirit, headman and healer; Stanley Looking Horse, pipe keeper and healer, and Vance Brings Pipe, singer and healer — sent a resolution to the United States Court of Claims objecting to a lawsuit being litigated in their name.

Sioux Nation of Indians v. United States of America is probably the longest running lawsuit in the history of American jurisprudence. Since it was filed in 1923, the lawsuit has always been, despite the opposition of the Lakota, about financial restitution — never about restoring the Black Hills to their rightful guardians. The point is, none of these Lakota witnesses ever counted for anything in the American judicial system: their pleas and objections were ignored for more than sixty years in federal court.

"The records show," Clifford says, that the tribes have consistently wanted the land back, but the attorneys have always said, 'That's fine, but that's impossible. We will get you the money instead.' For a hundred years, whenever the question came up, you can always find in the records that the Indians said, "We want the Black Hills back."

A GENERATION OF Washington lawyers grew old tending the case; when they died, a new generation took their place. In 1942, the case was dismissed on technical grounds, only to be reinstated eight years later. At last, in 1974, a claims commission set up by Congress awarded the Lakota $17.5 million for the Black Hills, plus $85 million in accumulated interest. The Justice Department objected to the payment of interest and appealed to the United States Court of Claims, which dismissed the claim on technical grounds even as it conceded, "A more ripe and rank case of dishonourable dealings will never, in all probability, be found in our history."

Finally, in 1980, an award of $105 million for the Black Hills was upheld by the Supreme Court. It was the largest Indian-claims settlement ever awarded, but it was not as magnanimous as it sounds. In 1923, the first lawyer for the tribes calculated their loss at $500 million in land, timber and minerals. In today's dollars, that's the equivalent of about $2.5 billion. According to one estimate, the Black Hills mines alone have yielded more than $2 billion in gold, not to mention uranium and other ores.

But even as they arrived at this settlement, the lawyers in Washington were hearing angry noises from their clients on the reservations. For years, the elected tribal governments had supported the litigation, but now they were under increasing pressure at home, both from traditional leaders and from young activists who wanted the tribes to reject the award and to pursue their original goal — the return of the Black Hills. One by one, the eight tribal councils passed resolutions refusing the settlement of their claim, demanding the land instead.

Caught in the middle, the Lakota's Washington lawyers went ahead and won the money. (They took ten percent of that — more than $10 million — in attorneys' fees.) In 1983, when the federal judge told the attorneys to visit the reservations and persuade their clients to take the claims money, the lawyers expressed some reluctance.

One lawyer, Marvin Sonosky, explained that on his last visit to Sioux country, angry crowds had run him off three reservations. "And now you want me to go back out into that country and sell them the same proposition because you put it down on paper?" Sonosky asked. "It cannot be done, and I owe it to my family not to expose myself to that kind of risk again."

Today lawyers on the case still shuffle papers and appear in court. The Lakota still will not accept the award. The money still accumulates interest in the Treasury Department. And *Sioux Nation of Indians v. United States of America* languishes in a legal limbo, a living monument to the mysteries of the white man's law.

CHARLOTTE BLACK ELK, a slender woman with large, serious eyes behind horn-rimmed glasses and gleaming long black hair, believes she was raised for this moment in history. She grew up in a canyon settlement called Manderson, a pocket of resistance where the clan of Crazy Horse settled after the Indian wars. When she was a girl, children in Manderson were still taught to speak Lakota and told the stories of the old faith.

Charlotte's long ago grandfathers include holy men and distinguished rebels — Hollow Horn, Plenty Wolf, Sun Dreamer, Black Elk. Hollow Horn performed a sun dance at Manderson in 1929 in defiance of the Indian agency; Black Elk became famous after he revealed to a white scholar the holy vision he received on Harney Peak in the Black Hills, which became the widely read book *Black Elk Speaks*.

Despite generations of repression, men organized as Those Who Speak of Sacred Things kept the secrets alive. As a child, Charlotte

Black Elk listened and remembered. "This activism has been a hundred years in the making," she says. "People knew exactly what they were doing. The elders taught us to get an education and learn to speak English better than the white people because, they said, 'Someday you're going to fight this battle.'

"The elders said to us, 'We lost one generation to the civilizers and the Christians. We lost another generation to the traumatic change and alcohol.' They said our generation would be the last — if we did not fight the battle — because the others would go the way of the drugs or choose not to be Lakota. This was the obligation placed on the grandchildren."

DESPITE WHAT THE court records in Washington show, the Lakota insist they were never willing to sell the Black Hills for money or to relinquish their sacred ground.

Charlotte's husband Gerald Clifford, 47, light-skinned, with long black hair, grew up on Pine Ridge, too, but he never learned to speak Lakota. Like Patrick Janis, he is a mixed blood, descended from an interpreter for chief Red Cloud who married into the tribe. His father was a coach at the Catholic mission school, and his mother wanted him to be a Catholic priest, but Clifford studied engineering and wound up designing missile components for an aerospace company in Los Angeles. Uncomfortable with urban culture and disgusted with what he was doing with his life, he retreated into his Catholic religion, living for six years under the stern rules of solitude and prayer at a monastery. Finally, it dawned on him: his search for spirituality ought to begin at home. Like many young Indians educated during the upheaval of the sixties, Clifford returned to the reservation. He began meeting with other young men who had returned to Pine Ridge and were now asking the same question: What does it mean to be an Indian?

"We essentially rejected the assimilation thing," he says. "We said to ourselves, 'It's good to be an Indian. We're going to be Lakota, whatever that is.' I found there was this tremendously rich spiritual heritage that I was part of by inheritance. I'd been kept from it. Now I had to learn it."

Clifford studied Lakota and learned to pray with the pipe, to fast and sweat, to call upon the spirits as his ancestors had done. And slowly he began to see a convergence between the Catholic and Lakota faiths in the figure of Jesus. "When the missionaries first came, Lakotas were very impressed with Jesus," he says. "They thought Jesus was a very good Lakota. He fasted on a mountaintop. He talked to the winds and the birds. He did the ultimate thing — dying so the people would live."

EQUIPPED WITH HIS seminary training, Clifford explored the theological principles embedded in the Lakota legends and discovered what set them apart from Christianity — and what was valuable in them for everyone.

"In the Judaeo-Christian origin story," he says, "God ousted Man from the garden and said that the earth would produce thorns and thistles and Man was going to have to work by the sweat of his brow to survive and he would have to dominate the earth, to subdue it. But the Lakota original story says that the earth is the mother who nourishes everything. It teaches respect for all living things, all related to one another. That's an important difference.

"When you look at what ails this society, the willingness to treat the earth as a commodity that can be used up, the Lakota have a lot to offer other people. What we do today is not for us alone; it's for our children and our children's children. What we do today must not dishonour our grandfathers. If we can bring people around to this theological principle — a way of thinking that is broader in time — it's going to benefit the entire society, not just the Lakota."

THE PRAIRIE IN winter appeared burned yellow, the colour of of straw, and empty as the open sea. Dusted with new snow, the grass glowed as though brushed by light. Driving across it alone, I briefly glimpsed what the Indians perhaps meant by their talk of the sacred earth. The empty landscape — rolling, dimpled prairie in every direction — first produced a moment of euphoria, the buoyancy of utter solitude. Against this endless land and sky, I felt small and insignificant.

In the distance I saw the Black Hills rising like a natural sanctuary over this harsh and humbling landscape: a few dozen miles north-west of Pine Ridge, the Black Hills hover over the vacant prairie like a dark green battlement. For generations, these hills were the sacred retreat of the Plains Indians. Even today, thousands of Lakota and Cheyenne return there each year seeking religious renewal. But now the Indians who undertake vision quests have to avoid the swarms of tourists visiting roadside attractions like the Life of Christ Wax Museum.

POLITICALLY, THE LAKOTA'S objective of regaining the Black Hills looks impossible. Owned mainly by the National Park Service and the

National Forest Service of the federal government, the Black Hills and their tourist attractions have become central to the commerce of western South Dakota. It takes an act of great faith to believe that the Congress of the United States of America would turn its back on the Flintstones merely to restore these sacred mountains to their rightful trustees.

One political leader who believes it can be done is Senator Bill Bradley of New Jersey, a practical, serious man who is hardly a romantic about the Indians or anything else. When he was playing for the New York Knickerbockers, Bradley conducted summer basketball clinics for the children of Pine Ridge, where he first heard the old stories about the Black Hills — about their sacred meaning and unjust theft. With Senator Daniel Inouye of Hawaii, he is co-sponsoring a bill, based on the recommendations of Gerald Clifford's Black Hills steering committee.

The measure would restore 1.3 million acres of land held by the federal government to the shared ownership of the Lakota tribes. It would establish a Sioux national park, owned by the Lakota and co-managed by the tribal governments and federal agencies. Neither privately held land nor federal installations such as Mount Rushmore would be disturbed. "This goes to the core of who we are as a people and what it means to be an American," Bradley says. "I am confident that over time justice will prevail."

It's only a beginning of course, but the legislation would be, as the senator calls it, "a new chapter". The young Lakota are trying to take what the old taught them and imagine a different future for their people, free of dependency on government handouts and responsible for their own lives. Enactment of the bill would not suddenly overcome generations of poverty, but it would fuse the practical with the spiritual. The Lakota would be compelled to work out their old differences and to manage the land wisely and well. At the same time, restoration of the land would restore their spiritual principles — a religion that promises its own healing powers for a people deeply wounded by history.

"Our relationships to one another as Lakota are defined by our relationship to the earth," Gerald Clifford says. "Until we get back on track in our relationship to the earth, we cannot straighten out any of our relationships to ourselves, to other people."

AND THE REST of America, if it listens closely, might even learn something about itself — about the mystery and the morality of our own relationship to the earth and about our history. Among the Lakota legends is a terrible prophecy that seems especially relevant to the nuclear age, a warning that mankind must reconcile itself to creation or some day face destruction. Charlotte Black Elk's great grandfather, John Hollow Horn, uttered the prophecy nearly sixty years ago when he danced the outlawed sun dance in Manderson: "A day will come in your life-time when the earth, your mother, will beg you, with tears running, to save her. Ho, if you fail to help her, you [the Lakota] and all people will die like dogs. Remember this."

ON A CHILL WINTER evening, Charlie Bear Robe stoked the huge bonfire in a back yard in the village of Pine Ridge. A cover of fresh snow encircled the fire, and Bear Robe poked at a heap of stones buried in the flames. One by one, as the stones glowed red-hot, Bear Robe removed them from the fire with a pitchfork and placed them inside a low-domed tent, the *ini tipi*. The tent was perfectly round, constructed with bent willow saplings in the way Lakota have always made the sweat lodge, only this one was covered with canvas tarpaulin instead of animal skins. A small altar of stones and forked sticks stood before the opening of the *ini tipi*, and as other people gathered by the fire, each one paused to place a small offering there.

Patrick Janis and the others began to disrobe discreetly in the cool night air. Tonight Janis would serve as the *eiyeska*, the interpreter who calls forth Inyan in the darkness of the sweat lodge, and perhaps hear from the spirits. "We pray to the rock spirits because we have lost confidence in our lives," Janis said. "We want to start over, to be born again. This is the womb of our mother; we go back into the womb and cast out all the bad things. When we come out, we are cleansed." By the firelight, the *ini tipi* did resemble the rounded belly of a pregnant woman rising from the earth.

WHEN ALL WERE huddled inside the sweat lodge, they became disembodied voices in the darkness, four men and six women squatting in a close circle around the glowing stones. Patrick's voice rose in a plaintive invocation, joined occasionally by murmured assents from the others.

"Grandfather, pity us," he called. "A lot of our people are in hard times. They are confused. They have problems that lead them to hurt one another. Pity them, Tunkasila. Take this water and purify them." A dipper of water was dashed on the hot stones, and steam filled the darkness — an intense bath of moist heat that pressed against one's breath and overwhelmed thought. Janis's invocation echoed a sweat-lodge prayer recorded on this reservation eighty years ago: "Sweat-lodge stones, pity me! Sun, pity me! Moon, pity me! Darkness of the night, pity me! Water, standing in a *wakan* manner, pity me! Grass, standing in the morning, pity me! Whatever pitiful one is scarcely able to crawl into the *tipi* and lie down for the night, see him and pity him."

Charlie Bear Robe sang a mournful, nasal chant, and Janis prayed again. Orville Looking Horse, a school-teacher, sang another Lakota hymn and was joined by the others. Led by Janis, the worshippers began a round of prayers, each one expressing whatever he or she felt most urgently. Four times, after each round of prayers, the tent flap was opened for a spell of coolness, then closed again. More water was offered to the stones, more overwhelming steam filled the darkness and erased the boundaries of self.

Their prayers were about elemental things: for the troubled children, for someone who was sick, for another whose father died. They asked the spirits to heal ailments and help the alcoholics, to comfort the lonely old people and see that they had firewood. Modest prayers, humble requests.

When the stones no longer glowed, the *ini tipi* became totally dark, a warm, floating void, strangely comforting. Janis announced the presence of spirits and spoke for them. As he talked, the black emptiness was punctuated by small sparkles of light, like miniature stars dancing among our voices. Even I could see them.

When the people emerged from the *ini tipi* into the cold night air, they felt cleansed and refreshed and once again whole.

Extracts from an article first published in **Rolling Stone**.

Published in *Resurgence* No. 124, September/October 1987.

Introduction to Peter Berg

BIOREGIONS

When I was at primary school, I used to write something in the front of my books — a ritual that many other children have carried out. It began with my name, my house number and my street and ended, 'The World, The Solar System, The Universe.' It reflected a desire common to us all; the desire to know where we are. Knowing where you are is part of knowing who you are, so that you can be yourself. Notions of personal identity are often linked to notions of place, as Snyder argues. So what are the appropriate ways of defining place?

  Peter Berg's article addresses this specific point. Like the two previous ones, it is about reinhabitation, which he defines as 'the practice of living-in-place', becoming part of a bioregion once again. 'Bioregion' is Berg's term for conceptualising a place in a way which takes heed of its biological, ecological, and climactic factors rather than by reference to a political map or something as abstract as lines of latitude. The importance of such bioregional definition is that it does justice to the natural processes which shape and characterise a particular location rather than follow the often arbitrary lines of political delineation.

The relevance of the bioregional concept to issues of health is not solely ecological, but is also shown in the experience of groups such as the Kurds or the Palestinians, who cannot easily find the names of their places on maps and who suffer in consequence, not least in their physical and mental health. The inappropriateness of proceeding by artificial straight-line boundaries is demonstrated by the Navajo, whose externally-defined homeland, 'dinetah', spreads across four of the United States of America. Significantly, as Dubos has shown, the Navajo can trace the loss of their former health status directly to specific intervention by the United States government.

Homeland is not a term that English people use easily. But in my homeland, the Wirral peninsula in the North-West of England, some of us have also been experimenting with the idea of the bioregion. We have been faced by ecological threats several times in the past few years through, for example, pollution of the sea, rivers, and the air. Fears of radiation, the importation of toxic waste, and of air pollution have been specific local issues in the last five years. To understand and to try to protect ourselves against such threats to our health we have been forced to think bioregionally.

For us, a logical way of conceptualising our bioregion has therefore been to think of it as the peninsula, the rivers Dee and Mersey that frame it, and the opposite banks of those two rivers — parts of North Wales and part of the Liverpool area. We have begun to speak of the Two Rivers bioregion. Identifying our bioregion helps us monitor, coordinate, and intervene when a problem seems imminent. Berg shows the relevance of bioregional thinking to health issues, for communities cannot be healthy if they are under ecological threat or experiencing actual damage. And bioregional thinking provides a context in which communities can cooperate to identify and oppose such threats.

FURTHER READING

Peter Berg, Beryl Magilavy & Seth Zuckerman (1991) **A Green City Program for the San Francisco Bay Area and Beyond**. Wingbow Press, USA.

Peter Berg (1991) **A Metamorphosis for Cities: from Gray to Green**. City Lights Journal, USA.

René Dubos (1960) **Mirage of Health**. George Allen & Unwin.

Mira Silva (1986) **Health and Development** in Paul Ekins (Ed) *The Living Economy*. Routledge, pp 21–28.

BIOREGIONS

PETER BERG

WHERE DO ANY OF US actually live? Since the advent of Industrial-Age consciousness only about two centuries ago (and for only the last few decades in most of the world) the answer to this literally basic question has been framed in progressively more urban, statist and technological terms, rather than in those of the processes of life itself. Ask the next person you meet and expect at least part of this reply, "In a numbered house on such a street, in some section of a city, in a particular state or province or department, of… nation-state, in a First, Second or Third World power bloc. That is, when I'm not at… another place where I commute to work by car, bus, train, or aeroplane."

We all live within the web-of-life, of course. Our bodies and senses are those of mammals in the biosphere. All of our food, water and materials comes from processes of the biosphere. But during the Industrial Age, reaching a climax in the Late Industrial period dating from World War II, the fact of our interdependence with all life became a vague abstraction. We have suffered from the delusion of believing that our lives were safely in the care of machines. The separation between conscious human identity and locatedness, and the planetary life-web of which our species is part, is now critical enough to threaten the survival of both. We are in the absurd and tragic position of someone who sets fire to the house to keep warm in a freezing blizzard, destroying ever-widening ranges of life without consciousness of our ultimate bond with them.

How do we rediscover where we actually live?

Bioregions are geographic areas having common characteristics of soil, watersheds, climate, and native plants and animals that exist within the whole planetary biosphere as unique and intrinsic contributive parts. Consider them as possessing the diverse and necessary distinction of leaves from roots, or arms from legs. The Amazon jungle, for instance, provides so much oxygen that it can be counted as a lung of the biosphere. The Nile delta is a kidney for the Mediterranean Sea. Underneath and around the industrial grids of row-houses and factories, streets and sewers, highways and railways, oil and gas pipe-lines, legal jurisdictions and political boundaries, this natural geography of life continues to endure.

Everyone lives in some bioregion or other. Prior to industrialism the reality of inhabitation in a unique life-place was reflected in adaptive cultures that reciprocated with cycles and conditions of that place. Some strong examples still remain such as the Hopi's deeply sacred involvement with arid cultivation of corn, rain, mesas, and respectful grace in the American South-west. Some vestiges continue to haunt the designs of nation-states such as the heroic persistence (after eight centuries' domination) of Welsh language and culture on the western side of England's principal topographical divide. Thoroughly adaptive cultures are native human mammal interactions, as natural as any other aspect of the life of a bioregion.

For most people, however, inhabitation of a unique bioregion has lost pre-eminence as a fact of survival. While this condition prevails no bioregion is secure from the threat of being crippled in its ability to nurture life. "Cut down the Amazon jungle for newspaper pulp — we need to read about fluctuations in oil prices." "Level the Hopi's Black Mesa — we need coal to produce electricity so Los Angeles' lights can burn all night." There is no way to ensure the survival of the biosphere without saving each bioregion, and it is especially important for anyone living within industrial society to begin cultivating bioregional consciousness.

Reinhabitation is a term for undertaking the practice of living-in-place, becoming part of a bioregion again. A first step is to become familiar with the specific natural characteristics of the place where one lives. Wet and green northern California, for example, isn't continuous with the dry desert portion of the state. Northern California is a separate natural country, "Shasta". The Ozark Mountains are a distinct raised limestone formation with a unique natural identity of watersheds and vegetation straddling the border of Arkansas and Missouri, the bioregion of "Ozarkia". Ocean-influenced areas of northern Maine in the United States and New Brunswick in Canada share the same bioregion, 'The Gulf of Maine'.

Any place is within a bioregion. Every metropolis exists in a natural locale: Manhattan in the lower Hudson River valley; London in that of the Thames. Suburbs, towns, villages, rural farming areas, forests and national parks are all within specific bioregions.

Once the extent and character of a life-place is determined, reinhabitory approaches can be taken to an impressively large number of activities and problem areas. Education and awareness have a special priority at present, and bioregional study groups have already emerged in over fifty areas of the United States and Canada. They produce newsletters and information "bundles" on their bioregions, and often choose particularly immediate political issues for emphasis. In Shasta, for example, the Frisco Bay Mussel Group evolved into an adamant voice for opposing interbasin transfers of northern California water to the south and Los Angeles, and in the 1982 election was active in defeating what up until now was a common practice (over 90% of Shasta voters opposed the latest diversion scheme; the largest single-side vote in Californian history).

For decentralists in general the concept of bioregion answers the question, "Decentralize to where?" Anti-nuclear activists are becoming pro-bioregionalist. Local food co-operatives and local natural resources defence groups are finding that organizing along watershed and bioregional lines makes them more effective.

Bioregionalism is a significant step beyond either conservationist or environmentalist thinking. It is directly addressed to the fate of the earth, not as merely an "ecological" issue, but as the central issue that human civilization must address.

*Peter Berg is editor of **Raise the Stakes** (The Planet Drum Review) and can be contacted at The Planet Drum Foundation, Box 31251, San Francisco, Shasta Bioregion, CA 94131, USA.*

Published in *Resurgence* No. 98, May/June 1983.

Introduction to Wendell Berry

HIGHER EDUCATION AND HOME DEFENCE

This section on *New Community Thinking* is opened by Wendell Berry. One of the memorable features of his piece is the notion of professional vandalism. This is what takes place when, in the attempt to serve the needs of society as a whole, the needs of many communities are disregarded by those who no longer belong to a community themselves.

You become a professional vandal when you lose your sense of place, Berry argues. First you go to College or University, but instead of returning home to carry back your learning for the enrichment of your community, you become a transient careerist. You lose the notion of anywhere as your home, and so lose a sensitivity to what it means for somewhere to be somebody else's. You are then ready to regard any place as a potential commodity, its specifics sacrificed for some general collective good.

Berry's home is in Kentucky and he writes from an American perspective, but I think his observations will strike chords in many European hearts as well. For me, the article elucidates three key issues of concern to healthy communities.

First is that the frequent assumption that 'leaving home' is the logical completion of growth to adult status must be questioned. Over the last century the development of higher (and yet higher) education has tended to produce a migration of the young — they leave home for Higher Education and then take up work where they were trained or move to wherever the work can be found. This is eminently understand-able, but in consequence a community's richest resource — the energy and intelligence of its next generation — is dissipated rather than returned to enrich and regenerate that community. The development of distance learning techniques and the growing awareness of the impor-tance of community living may modify this trend in the future.

Second, Berry's piece underscores the adage about thinking globally but acting locally. Only local people — people committed to the community — can be trusted to address and solve community problems in ways that identify real issues and produce genuine solutions, rather than 'technical fixes' or a cosmetic gloss on a problem that persists. This is not to deny the importance of expertise; we should not forget the community that passed a law making the mathematical constant pi exactly equal to three "to save time in school". But if the expertise is home-grown it will be far more sympathetic and far more likely to be a source of good advice. It is also more likely to be refusable — many community action groups have discovered the wisdom of having experts on tap, not on top!

Finally, Berry's work is a reminder about the importance of choosing sides. This century the conflict between the powerful, international expert whose solutions allegedly help everyone in general but no one in particular and the besieged community desperate to defend its own place, school, shops, quality of life or even physical existence has become ever more acute. And a consequence of people choosing the right side is that communities become progressively empowered, they regenerate, and in rediscovering our communities we rediscover our true social selves. This is why community development is an important and growing mode of action in health promotion, and why it needs to be fostered and developed.

FURTHER READING

Trieste Kennedy & Maria Rodale **Community Options**. The Regeneration Project, 33 E. Minor St., Emmaus, PA 18098, USA.

John Tyme (1982) **Motorways versus Democracy**. Published by author.

Des Wilson (1986) **Citizen Action — Taking action in your community**. Longman.

HIGHER EDUCATION
AND HOME DEFENCE

WENDELL BERRY

S EVERAL YEARS AGO, I attended a meeting at Madison, Indiana, that I have been unable to forget, it seems to be emblematic of the fate of our country in our time. In the audience at that meeting were many citizens of local communities — my own among them — who were mistrustful and afraid of the nuclear power plant then, and still, being built at Marble Hill. Seated on the stage were representatives of Public Service Indiana, which was building the power plant, and members of the Nuclear Regulatory Commission, whose job it presumably was to protect us from the acknowledged dangers of the use of nuclear power, as well as from the already recognized deceits and ineptitude of Public Service Indiana.

The meeting proceeded as such meetings typically proceed. The fears, objections, questions, and complaints of the local people were met with technical jargon and with bland assurances that the chance of catastrophe was small. In such a confrontation, the official assumption apparently is that those who speak most incomprehensibly and dispassionately are right; and that those who speak plainly and with feeling are wrong. Local allegiances, personal loyalties, and private fears are not scientifically respectable; they do not weigh at all against "objective consideration of the facts" — even though some of the "facts" may be highly speculative, or false. And indeed in the history of such confrontations, the victories have mainly gone to the objective considerers of the so-called facts.

They are still winning at Marble Hill, even though the fraud and incompetence of Public Service Indiana is more a matter of public record now than it was then. But that meeting produced one question and one answer which should tell us all we need to know about the nature of that victory, and more than we like to know about the role of

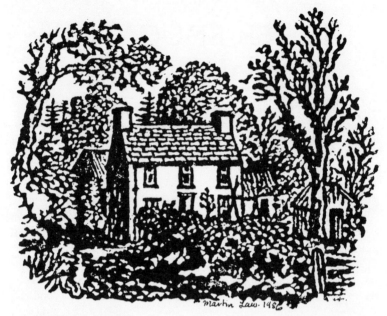

Illustration by Martin Law

education in such an enterprise. A lady rose in the audience and asked the fifteen or twenty personages on the stage to tell us how many of them lived within the fifty-mile danger zone around Marble Hill. The question proved tactically brilliant, apparently shocking to the personages on the stage, who were forced to give it the shortest, plainest answer of the evening: *Not one.* Not a single one of those well-paid, well-educated, successful, important men would need to worry about his family or his property in the event of a catastrophic mistake at Marble Hill.

THIS STORY WOULD have no point beyond the Marble Hill danger zone if it was unusual. My point, of course, is that it is *not* unusual. Some version of it is now happening in this country virtually everywhere, virtually every day. Everywhere, every day local life is being discomforted, disrupted, endangered or destroyed by powerful people who live, or who are privileged to think that they live, beyond the bad effects of their bad work.

A powerful class of itinerant professional vandals is now pillaging the country and laying it waste. Their vandalism is not called by that name because of its enormous profitability (to some) and the grandeur of its scale. If one wrecks a private home, *that* is vandalism. But if, to build a nuclear power plant, one destroys good farmland, disrupts a local community, and jeopardizes lives, homes, and properties within an area of several thousand square miles, *that* is industrial progress.

For membership in this prestigious class of rampaging professionals, there are two requirements.

The first requirement is that they must be careerists — transients, at least in spirit. That is, they must have no local allegiances; they must not have a local point-of-view. In order to be able to desecrate, endanger, or destroy a *place*, after all, one must be able to leave it and forget it. One must never think of any place as one's *home*. One must never think of any place as anyone else's home. One must believe that no place is as valuable as what it might be changed into, or as what might be got out of it. Unlike a life at home, which makes ever more particular and precious the places and creatures of this world, the careerist's life generalizes the world, reduces its abounding and comely diversity to "raw material".

When education institutions educate people to *leave* home, then they have re-defined education as "career preparation". In doing so, they have made it a commodity — something to be *bought* to make money with. The great wrong in this is that it obscures the fact that education — real education — is free. I am necessarily well aware that schools and books have a cost that must be paid, but I am sure nevertheless that what is taught and learned is free. None of us would be so foolish as to suppose that the worth of a good book is the same as the money value of its paper and ink, or that the worth of a good teacher is equal to his or her salary. What is taught and learned is free. Priceless, but free. To make a commodity of it is to work its ruin, for when we put a price on it, we both reduce its value and blind the recipient to the obligations that always accompany good gifts: to use them well, and to hand them on unimpaired.

To make a commodity of education, then, is inevitably to make a kind of weapon of it — to dissociate it from the sense of obligation, and so to put it directly at the service of greed.

THE PEOPLE ON the stage at the meeting I began by describing no doubt thought of themselves as "public servants". But they were servants of the *general* public, which means, in practice, that they might be enemies at any time to any particular segment of that general public. As servants of what they would have thought of as the general good, they stood ready to sacrifice the good of any particular community or place — which, of course, is a way of saying that they had no reliable way to distinguish between the public interest and their own. When they appeared before us, they were serving their own professional commitment and their own ambition. They had not come to reassure us so far as they honestly could do so, or to redress our just grievances. They had not come even to determine if our grievances were just. They had come to mislead us, to bewilder us with the jargon of their expertise, to imply that our fears were ignorant and selfish. Their manner of paying attention to us was simply a way of ignoring us.

That meeting, then, was not really a meeting at all, but one of the enactments of a division that is rapidly deepening in our country: a division between people who are trying to defend the health, the integrity, even the existence of places whose values they sum up in the words "home" and "community", and people for whom those words signify no value at all. I do not hesitate to say — what I strongly feel — that right is on the side of the defenders of homes and communities.

I do not mean to say that people with local allegiances and local

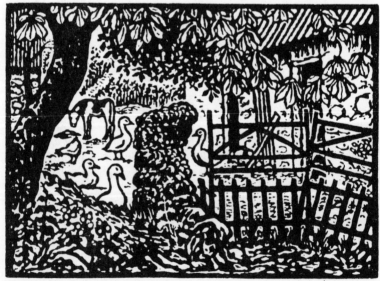

Illustration by Martin Law

points of view would have no legitimate interest in energy. I do mean to say that their interest would be different in both quality and kind from the present *professional* interest. They could not willingly use energy that destroyed its natural or human source, or that endangered the user or the place of use. They would not believe that they could improve their neighbourhoods by making them unhealthy or dangerous. They would not believe that it could be necessary to destroy their community in order to save it.

The second requirement for entrance into the class of professional vandals is "higher education". One's eligibility must be certified by a college, for whatever the real condition or quality of the minds in it, this class is both intellectual and elitist. It proposes to do its vandalism by *thinking*; insofar as its purposes will require dirty hands, *other* hands will be employed.

MANY OF THESE professionals have been educated, at considerable public expense, in colleges or universities that had originally a clear mandate to serve localities or regions — to receive the daughters and sons of their regions, educate them, and send them home again to serve and strengthen their communities. The outcome shows, I think, that they have generally betrayed this mandate, having worked instead to uproot the best brains and talents, to direct them away from home into exploitative careers, and so to make them predators of communities and homelands, their own and other people's.

Education in the true sense, of course, is an enablement to *serve* both the living human community in its natural household or neighbourhood and the precious cultural possessions that the living community inherits or should inherit. To educate is, literally, to "bring up", to bring young people to a responsible maturity, to help them to be good caretakers of what they have been given, to help them to be charitable toward fellow creatures. Such an education is obviously pleasant and useful to have. That a sizeable number of humans should have it is probably also one of the necessities of human life in this world. If this education is to be used well, it is obvious that it must be used some*where*; it must be used where one lives, where one intends to continue to live; it must be brought home.

Wendell Berry is a farmer and writer who lives in Kentucky.

Published under the title "Defending Our Homes and Communities" in *Resurgence* No. 123, July/August 1987.

PART TWO

NEW COMMUNITY THINKING

Introduction to Wendell Berry

WORD AND FLESH

It is appropriate that one of Berry's pieces should end the first section and another begin the second. What Berry does in this article is to demonstrate the practical links between the movement towards re-inhabitation and the development of ways of living appropriate to a healthy community.

He explores the contradictions inherent in the notion of global thinking. The problem with what is presented as global thinking, Berry suggests, is that it can cultivate the false belief that any one of us can save the planet. This is absurd — to imagine that a single person could save a planet is to indulge in fantasy.

But what we can do is to try to save our own place. I cannot hope to save the world; but I can try to help save Hooton, which is my place. The same is true for all the rest of us. And this, Berry argues, is in reality how the world gets saved — by all of us embodying our care for the environment by caring for the human and natural communities which we inhabit in practice. This is how we achieve the care of 'the planet's millions of human and natural neighbourhoods'.

So rather than becoming what his previous piece termed professional vandals, we build a healthy planet by building a healthy community. Berry describes the building blocks through which this can be accomplished. Deriving from a commencement address, they can well serve as six pointers to a healthy and sustainable community:

- Make a home   • Put the community first
- Love your neighbours   • Love this miraculous world
- Make your life dependent on your local place
- Find work that does no damage — and enjoy it

Simple advice; but possibly worth more than many multi-million pound research projects. And, like the rest of this article, a clear and pragmatic indication of the nature of the relationship between a healthy community and a healthy planet. It may sometimes be appropriate to think globally, but the importance of committed local action must never be understated. Human problems almost always require human-scale solutions. Conversely, large scale solutions almost always make life worse for those who were supposed to benefit. These are important lessons for anyone in the health business.

WORD AND FLESH

WENDELL BERRY

T OWARD THE END of Shakespeare's play *As You Like It*, Orlando says, "I can live no longer by thinking." He is ready to marry Rosalind. It is time for incarnation. Having thought too much, he is at one of the limits of human experience, or of human sanity. If his love does put on flesh, we know he must sooner or later arrive at the opposite limit, at which he will say, "I can live no longer without thinking." Thought — even consciousness — seems to live between these limits: the abstract and the particular, the word and the flesh.

All public movements of thought quickly produce a language that works as a code, useless to the extent that it is abstract. It is readily evident, for example, that you can't conduct a relationship with another person in terms of the rhetoric of the civil rights movement or the women's movement — as useful as those rhetorics may initially have been to personal relationships.

The same is true of the environment movement. The favourite adjective of this movement now seems to be *planetary*. This word is used, properly enough, to refer to the interdependence of places, and to the recognition, which is desirable and growing, that no place on the earth can be completely healthy until all places are.

But the word *planetary* also refers to an abstract anxiety or an abstract passion that is desperate and useless exactly to the extent that it is abstract. How, after all, can anybody, any particular body, do anything to heal a planet? Nobody can do anything to heal a planet. The suggestion that anybody could do so is preposterous. The heroes of abstraction keep galloping in on their white horses to save the planet, and they keep falling off in front of the grandstand.

What we need, obviously, is a more intelligent — which is to say, a more accurate — description of the problem. The description of a problem as planetary arouses a motivation for which, of necessity, there is no employment. The adjective *planetary* describes a problem in such a way that it cannot be solved. In fact, though we now have serious problems nearly everywhere on the planet, we have no problem that can accurately be described as planetary. And, short of the total annihilation of the human race, there is no planetary solution.

There are also no national, state, or county problems, and no national, state, or county solutions. That will-o'-the-wisp, the large-scale solution to the large-scale problem, which is so dear to governments, universities, and corporations, serves mostly to distract people from the small, private problems that they may, in fact, have the power to solve.

The problems, if we describe them accurately, are all private and small. Or they are so initially.

The problems are our lives. In the "developed" countries, at least, the large problems occur because all of us are living either partly wrongly or almost entirely wrongly. It was not just the greed of corporate shareholders and the hubris of corporate executives that put the fate of Prince William Sound into one ship; it was also our demand that energy be cheap and plentiful.

The economies of our communities and households are wrong. The answers to the human problems of ecology are to be found in economy. And the answers to the problems of economy are to be found in culture and in character. To fail to see this is to go on dividing the world falsely between guilty producers and innocent consumers.

The planetary versions — the heroic versions — of our problems have attracted great intelligence. Our problems, as they are caused and suffered in our lives, our households, and our communities, have attracted very little intelligence.

There are some notable exceptions. A few people have learned to do a few things better. But it is discouraging to reflect that, though we have been talking about most of our problems for decades, we are still mainly *talking* about them. The civil rights movement has not given us better communities. The women's movement has not given us better marriages or better households. The environment movement has not changed our parasite relationship to nature.

WE HAVE FAILED to produce new examples of good home and community economies, and we have nearly completed the destruction of the examples we once had. Without examples, we are left with theory and the bureaucracy and the meddling that come with theory. We change our principles, our thoughts, and our words, but these are changes made in the air. Our lives go on unchanged.

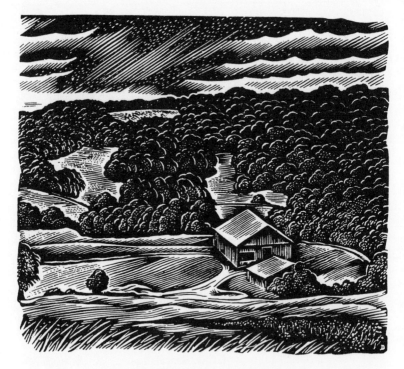

For the most part, the subcultures, the countercultures, the dissent-
ers, and the opponents continue mindlessly — or perhaps just helplessly
— to follow the pattern of the dominant society in its extravagance, its
wastefulness, its dependencies, and its addictions. The old problem
remains: How do you get intelligence *out* of an institution or an
organization?

My small community in Kentucky has lived and dwindled for a
century at least under the influence of four kinds of organization:
governments, corporations, schools, and churches — all of which are
distant (either actually or in interest), centralized, and consequently
abstract in their concerns.

Governments and corporations (except for employees) have no
presence in our community at all, which is perhaps fortunate for us, but
we nevertheless feel the indifference or the contempt of governments
and corporations for communities such as ours.

We have had no school of our own for nearly thirty years. The
school system takes our young people, prepares them for "the world of

tomorrow", which it does not expect to take place in any rural area, and gives back expert (that is, extremely generalized) ideas.

The church is present in the town. We have two churches. But both have been used by their denominations, for almost a century, to provide training and income for student ministers, who do not stay long enough even to become disillusioned.

For a long time, then, the minds that have most influenced our town have not been *of* the town and so have not tried even to perceive, much less to honour, the good possibilities that are there. They have not wondered on what terms a good and conserving life might be lived there. In this, my community is not unique but is like almost every other neighbourhood in our country and in the "developed" world.

The question that *must* be addressed, therefore, is not how to care for the planet but how to care for each of the planet's millions of human and natural neighbourhoods, each of its millions of small pieces and parcels of land, each one of which is in some precious way different from all the others. Our understandable wish to preserve the planet must somehow be reduced to the scale of our competence — that is, to the wish to preserve all of its humble households and neighbourhoods.

What can accomplish this reduction? I will say again, without

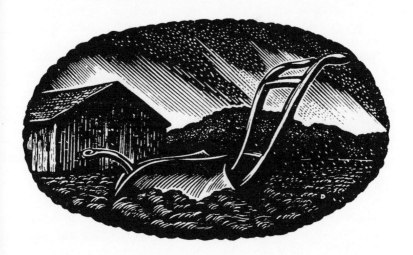

Wood engravings by Jon de Pol from Wendell Berry's book of poetry "Traveling at Home" (North Point Press)

overweening hope but with certainty nonetheless, that only love can do it. Only love can bring intelligence out of the institutions and organizations, where it aggrandizes itself, into the presence of the work that must be done.

Love is never abstract. It does not adhere to the universe or the planet or the nation or the institution or the profession but to the singular sparrows of the street, the lilies of the field, "the least of these my brethren". Love is not, by its own desire, heroic. It is heroic only when compelled to be. It exists by its willingness to be anonymous, humble, and unrewarded.

The older love becomes, the more clearly it understands its involvement in partiality, imperfection, suffering, and mortality. Even so, it longs for incarnation. It can live no longer by thinking.

And yet to put on flesh and do the flesh's work, it must think.

IN HIS ESSAY on Kipling, George Orwell wrote: "All left-wing parties in the highly industrialized countries are at bottom a sham, because they make it their business to fight against something which they do not really wish to destroy. They have internationalist aims, and at the same time they struggle to keep up a standard of life with which those aims are incompatible. We all live by robbing Asiatic coolies, and those of us who are "enlightened" all maintain that those coolies ought to be set free; but our standard of living, and hence our "enlightenment", demands that the robbery shall continue."

This statement of Orwell's is clearly applicable to our situation now; all we need to do is change a few nouns. The religion and the environmentalism of the highly industrialized countries are at bottom a sham, because they make it their business to fight against something that they do not really wish to destroy. We all live by robbing nature, but our standard of living demands that the robbery shall continue.

We must achieve the character and acquire the skills to live much poorer than we do. We must waste less. We must do more for ourselves and each other. It is either that or continue merely to think and talk about changes that we are inviting catastrophe to make.

The great obstacle is simply this: the conviction that we cannot change because we are dependent upon what is wrong. But that is the addict's excuse, and we know that it will not do.

How dependent, in fact, are we? How dependent are our neighbourhoods and communities? How might our dependences be reduced? To answer these questions will require better thoughts and better deeds than we have been capable of so far.

We must have the sense and the courage, for example, to see that the ability to transport food for hundreds or thousands of miles does not necessarily mean that we are well off. It means that the food supply is more vulnerable and more costly than a local food supply would be. It means that consumers do not control or influence the healthfulness of their food supply and that they are at the mercy of the people who have the control and influence. It means that, in eating, people are using large quantities of petroleum that other people in another time are almost certain to need.

I am trying not to mislead you, or myself, about our situation. I think that we have hardly begun to realize the gravity of the mess we are in.

OUR MOST SERIOUS problem, perhaps, is that we have become a nation of fantasists. We believe, apparently, in the infinite availability of finite resources. We persist in land-use methods that reduce the potentially infinite power of soil fertility to a finite quantity, which we then proceed to waste as if it were an infinite quantity. We have an economy that depends not upon the quality and quantity of necessary goods and services but on the behaviour of a few stockbrokers. We believe that democratic freedom can be preserved by people ignorant of the history of democracy and indifferent to the responsibilities of freedom.

Our leaders have been for many years as oblivious to the realities and dangers of their time as were George III and Lord North. They believe that the difference between war and peace is still the overriding political difference — when, in fact, the difference has diminished to the point of insignificance. How would you describe the difference between modern war and modern industry — between, say, bombing and strip mining, or between chemical warfare and chemical manufacturing? The difference seems to be only that in war the victimization of humans is directly intentional and in industry it is "accepted" as a "trade-off".

Were the catastrophes of Love Canal, Bhopal, Chernobyl, and the *Exxon Valdez* episodes of war or of peace? They were, in fact, peace-time acts of aggression, intentional to the extent that the risks were known and ignored.

We are involved unremittingly in a war not against "foreign en-emies" but against the world, against our freedom, and indeed against our existence. Our so-called industrial accidents should be looked upon as revenges of Nature. We forget that Nature is necessarily party to all our enterprises and that she imposes conditions of her own.

Now she is plainly saying to us, "If you put the fates of whole communities or cities or regions or ecosystems at risk in single ships or factories or power plants, then I will furnish the drunk or the fool or the imbecile who will make the necessary small mistake."

And so, graduates, my advice to you is simply my hope for us all:

Beware the justice of Nature.

Understand that there can be no successful human economy apart from Nature or in defiance of Nature.

Understand that no amount of education can overcome the innate limits of human intelligence and responsibility. We are not smart enough or conscious enough or alert enough to work responsibly on a gigantic scale.

In making things always bigger and more centralized, we make them both more vulnerable in themselves and more dangerous to everything else. Learn, therefore, to prefer small-scale elegance and generosity to large-scale greed, crudity, and glamour.

Make a home. Help to make a community. Be loyal to what you have made.

Put the interest of the community first.

Love your neighbours — not the neighbours you pick out, but the ones you have.

Love this miraculous world that we did not make, that is a gift to us.

As far as you are able, make your lives dependent upon your local place, neighbourhood, and household — which thrive by care and generosity — and independent of the industrial economy, which thrives by damage.

Find work, if you can, that does no damage. Enjoy your work. Work well.

Adapted from a commencement address given at the College of the Atlantic in Bar Harbor, Maine.

Published under the title "The Futility of Global Thinking" in *Resurgence* No. 139, March/April 1990.

Introduction to Barry Cooper

UNDERSTANDING BUREAUCRACY

The story so far has included a strong argument for decentralisation; the contention that we must return to home and some sense of place if we are to be mentally and physically healthy. Such a process involves attempting to solve planetary problems by addressing them at the level of community intervention and thus having some chance of success. Many argue that progressive decentralisation — a systematic unplugging of individuals and their communities from global power systems, global economics, global agriculture — is the only way in which we can make the transition to a sustainable human presence on the earth. Decentralisation is seen a prerequisite of local and thence global health and well-being.

But decentralisation is not a panacea; it presents a number of difficulties which have to be faced and overcome. You cannot decentralise unless there is some meaningful local community organisation to which you can decentralise. And it is difficult to decentralise if there is a major bureaucratic structure which is determined to proceed in precisely the opposite direction.

So bureaucracy is an opponent of decentralisation, and on the grounds of knowing the enemy this piece by Barry Cooper comes next. Cooper offers an insightful analysis of bureaucracies, and indicates some of their key features.

Bureaucracies can have two great deficiencies — they can be unimaginative, and they can be disempowering. In their desire to meet equal need with equal provision they produce plans and schemes which are uniformly grey and standard; reducing rather than celebrating differences between regions and communities. In their hierarchical structure, which Weber described many years ago, they inhibit the development of grassroots community initiatives. Of course, bureaucrats argue against decentralisation because they contend that only a small amount of any public money is spent on central staff. What this argument ignores, as Cooper points out, is that with decentralisation comes the elimination of many time- and money-wasting bureaucratic procedures. It can also produce people passionately committed to their work because its relevance is immediately discernable. The decentralist argument is that this could result in teachers having time to teach, nurses having time to spend with patients, and police spending time on the streets.

But the jury may still be out on bureaucracy. Cooper's critique rings true for many large organisations, but in recent years modern management theory has attempted to meet some of these objections by a recognition of the drawbacks of classical bureaucracy. Many commercial organisations have discovered for themselves that classical bureaucracy does not produce the best results. There is something called new management, which is empowering rather than directing, with fewer managerial layers. It employs matrix management and group working to build quality cultures where, it is said, each individual is encouraged to contribute to goal setting and to building success. The success rates of organisations adopting the new paradigm are variable, and it can be argued that these techniques require managers of such high calibre that they could probably make unreconstructed bureaucracy work just as well.

But it would be good to think that large bureaucracies could be made more human and more responsive. As well as being bad for the health of those they try to serve, they are also undoubtedly bad for the health of those who work within them. Poor management produces inappropriate levels of stress; and such stress is directly implicated not only in specific diseases such as Coronary Heart Disease (CHD) but also in a general inhibition of the body's immune system. Stress is also implicated in depression and anxiety.

The Ottawa Charter on Health Promotion identified three skills in health promoters — advocacy, mediation, and empowerment. It could be argued that a complex, centralised bureaucracy militates against all three. Bureaucracies disempower — they stifle imagination and initiative at community level. They do not mediate — rather they impose decisions on a community and then fight that community's resistance with funds obtained by taxing the community. Rather than facilitate advocacy, their complex procedural and legal processes make it well nigh impossible for an ordinary person to represent his or her views effectively.

All this gets in the way of community development, as Cooper graphically illustrates with his examples of the village school — often regarded as a linchpin of community life but increasingly threatened by bureaucracy. Decentralisation is a significant element in the growth and maintenance of a healthy community; bureaucracy may be one of its biggest impediments.

FURTHER READING

Eileen Conn (1991) **The Ecological Organisation: A New Perspective**. *Management Education and Development* Vol 22 Part 3, pp 227–233.

Cary Cooper (1988) **Causes, Coping and Consequences of Stress at Work**. Wiley.

Ivan Illich (1975) **Tools for Conviviality**. Fontana / Collins.

UNDERSTANDING
BUREAUCRACY

BARRY COOPER

**Those who believe in decentralization and work within bu-
reaucracies have a special understanding of what we are all
up against. It is important that there is a wider understanding of how bureaucracies work if there is to be a better
chance of reversing the centralist trends. The only way to
achieve decentralization is to dismantle the bureaucracies**.

I F DECENTRALIZATION is to be made to work there are some
hard truths to be faced up to. Ironically it may be that we can work
best for decentralization by learning about bureaucratic thinking
— because, almost always, decentralization means doing the opposite of
what a bureaucrat would do.

One important thing to realize about bureaucrats is that with very
few exceptions their power and salaries are directly related to the size of
their empires. So it is quite natural that they always seek to employ
more and more staff, which in turn leads to more administrative
centralization. Individuals should not be criticized for behaving like this
— the bureaucratic system dictates that this is the way to advance their
careers.

The way bureaucrats work is to establish administrative and pseudo-
technical processes which enable them to determine what services are
"needed". To be able to do this in a way that they see to be fair they
have to adopt a philosophy in which the aim is to provide equal services
in equal circumstances. Needless to say this aim is rarely achieved but it
is the main plank on which bureaucracy is based — take it away and
there is muddle. Much of the day-to-day muddle that we notice,
particularly in local government, is where politicians have rejected the
advice of their bureaucrats and together they then flounder together

from one bit of nonsense to the next.

The pseudo-technical processes invented by bureaucrats becomes incredibly complicated as the bureaucracies themselves become bigger. One example of this is transportation planning. The idea is to set standards of road and public transport provision, to pose alternative plans to achieve these standards and then to go through sophisticated evaluation processes to enable a "preferred" plan to be chosen. The chosen plan is usually too expensive to implement and so in due course the whole rigmarole has to be repeated to find a plan which can be afforded. In recent years the process has been lengthened by so-called "public participation" which is supposed to enable the objectives the bureaucrats have set on behalf of the community to be "weighted" towards what they think the public want. This does not mean, of course, that the solutions are any more likely to be what people really want.

The outcome is well-known. New roads and "improvement" schemes which impose high social costs locally are built because "on balance" they are said to be in the interests of the whole community. The local social costs are not included in the financial cost of road-building. If they were, fewer roads would have been built — and local people would have been properly compensated when roads were built.

Throughout the process there is a constant assumption — that in equal situations individual people will behave according to the way "Mr Average-man" is perceived to behave. What other assumption could a bureaucrat make and still see himself to be acting in a reasonable manner?

It is not surprising therefore that what emanates from bureaucracies is a constant greyness. Roads look the same with the same street lights and other furniture. There are almost identical housing estates throughout the country. Even our villages are beginning to become standardized.

The whole process is reinforced by the constant movement of staff between bureaucracies — being the quickest way up the promotion ladder. The Civil Service under successive governments are progressively applying national standards to just about everything. The professions set exams in which a knowledge of standards and processes is all-important. Inevitably the result is sameness throughout the country.

A tiny example of all this, showing how far things have gone, is the regulations for licensed minibuses. They all have to carry at least two stainless steel safety pins in their first-aid boxes!

This example illustrates another feature of bureaucracies, namely the

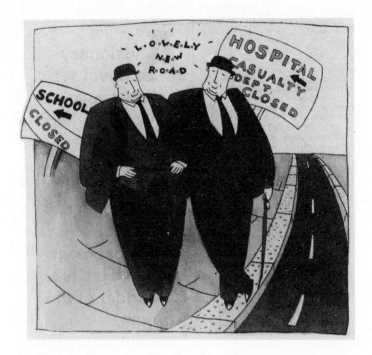

Illustration by Sarah-Jane Smith

minimization of risks. At first sight, this is a very reasonable attitude for bureaucrats to take — who would disagree that minibuses should be made as safe as possible? The safety pins are just one aspect of a whole range of requirements with the result that minibuses are much more expensive to run and fewer people can afford to use them. This means that people will either have fewer travel opportunities or, if they choose to cycle or walk, they face even greater risks of injury or death. So apparently reasonable safety standards, which are prescribed in the public interest, may well have quite the opposite effect to that intended.

This effect can be seen in every sphere of life where there is centralist involvement. Where a public service is being provided a monopoly situation is created so that very often it is impossible for people to choose what they want — they must have the service that is offered, or go without.

Decisions on rural bus services are almost always taken by County

Hall and Nationalized Bus Company bureaucrats. Their decisions are reinforced on the ground by the licensing legislation administered by the Traffic Commissioners which ensures that it is difficult, usually impossible, for other transport services to be provided. As a result even if a village wants to run its own minibus service, it is impossible without the backing of the bureaucrats.

The outcome — and this applies to most public services — is that local ideas and initiatives are stifled.

In reality individual people and villages have a diverse range of wants which are rarely met by the services imposed by bureaucracy. People either get more or less than they want — hardly good value for public money spent.

The centralists' answer is to strive to increase the services provided so that more and more people get what they want. For more services to be provided the Administration has to grow and so bureaucratic empires and power increase.

One centralist argument against decentralization is that it will not save money because only a small proportion of public expenditure is on central staff. It is said that setting up numerous small authorities would be inefficient because the total number of staff required would be even greater. This argument shows no understanding of what decentralization means. It means amongst other things, that the administrative processes, designed to minimize the risks to individual bureaucrats, would be abandoned. As a result public employees at the "point of service" — social workers, highway engineers, medical staff in hospitals — would be able to devote all their time to helping people get the services they want, instead of spending time "pushing paper" around for the bureaucrats.

Public money would then be well spent, because it would be used to give local people what they want, instead of being wasted on attempting to provide the same services for everyone, irrespective of whether they are wanted or not. Also, it would mean that the number of public purses could be reduced. The nonsense of money being spent on bringing local roads "up to standard" when at the same time there is no money available to provide staff at a cottage hospital could no longer happen.

Reductions in public expenditure in rural areas seem to be inevitable. The main British political parties seem to want to put an increasing share of public money into the big cities. This must mean that less public money will be spent in rural areas. In these areas the case for decentralization is getting stronger because it would ensure that the best value is gained from what little money is available.

Of course the growth of bureaucracy in the small authorities, resulting from decentralization, would have to be resisted. But that should be much easier than has been found possible with large remote organizations which are much more able to defend themselves.

Another feature of centralization is that a new language has evolved which is completely incomprehensible to anyone not "in the know". Most people are aware of the excessive use of jargon but the insidious perversion of day-to-day language is less obvious. It has happened without those "inside" or "outside" bureaucracies being aware of it.

Outsiders who talk of planning their lives mean making arrangements beforehand. Insiders see planning as the production of documents such as their corporate plans — plans which seek to organize people's lifestyle and environment in ways seen by insiders to be best for the community "at large". Co-ordination to a bureaucrat means organizing things from the centre; to a villager it means getting together with other people so that everyone benefits from mutual help. Everyone takes risks in one's day-to-day life, an awareness of the risks determines what people do. They know that to succeed they have to take risks. A centralist does everything possible to minimize risks. Risks are part of life in the "everyday" world, but a risk is like a dirty word to a bureaucrat.

The question then is how can things be changed? What has to happen to force decentralization to occur?

At first sight it may be thought that reorganization of the public services is all that is needed. But, for this to work there have to bureaucrats within the system who believe in decentralization and understand what is required, working alongside politicians who also understand. This is too fantastic to be possible. Whoever heard of senior public servants wanting to dismantle their bureaucracies?

Attitudes and beliefs have to change before we can progress towards decentralization. The most important step in that direction is not to reorganize the system but to arbitrarily and progressively reduce the number of central administrators. The extent and rate of the reduction would have to be arbitrary because there is no logical way to determine what would be best. Progress can be made with quite simple decisions that do not necessarily require a political commitment to decentralization at the outset. Commitment would come as the outcome becomes evident — gradual decentralization — and is seen to be what people want.

Once the public authorities realized that they have to manage with fewer and fewer central staff decentralization would "naturally" begin to creep in as they found ways to cope. Government Departments would be unable to send as many circulars out to public authorities and businesses. Services such as hospitals would soon learn how to run themselves without directives from the centre. County and District Councils, unable to deal with their work in the "old" ways would have to look more and more to the Parish Councils to decide how money should be spent. Social workers, highway maintenance engineers, doctors, bus operators, headmasters, would all find that their future depended on working closely with the new decision makers at the "grass roots".

This could happen without any changes in the law or reorganization of the public authorities.

A decision to reduce the bureaucracy could be taken separately from what is perhaps a more contentious political issue — whether there should be more or less public authority expenditure. If spending levels stay the same, then those who believe in decentralization would expect public services to improve. If there were less public expenditure, then services would not deteriorate in the way they would with centralization.

The only losers would be the bureaucrats who choose to stay and would have to put up with diminishing empires and power, although they may have more job satisfaction. On the ground — in day-to-day life — the changes would soon become noticeable. Unlike the creeping centralization, of the last fifty years or more, which most people have hardly noticed, a change of direction would be very evident. Day-to-day decisions, which had previously moved things towards centralization, would move in the opposite direction. The options that bureaucrats now pose to the politicians as being the only feasible ones all have an underlying theme — to find the best way to move towards centralization. The choice between moving towards or away from centralization is not posed. Once the bureau-empires being to shrink, the natural question each time a decision has to be taken, will be, what is the best way to decentralize. The result will be that most of the decisions will be the opposite of those taken now — an opposite which is not even considered today.

Take an example of the schools.

A County Council has to decide what to do about a small village school. After a period of uncertainty and what the media call "reprievals" the centralists will close the school and concentrate expenditure on schools in the nearest town and sending village children to them by bus. It is argued that the bigger town schools can give a wider education with more specialist subjects being taught. In a new climate of shrinking bureaucracy the Education Department would be less able to control things like catchment areas and school transport and they would be unable to keep separate "pockets" of money for distribution to the schools. The County Architects Department would not have staff to design and supervise improvements to school buildings. The County Treasurer's Department would not have accountants and clerks to pay salaries and bills or man the computer. There would not be enough administrators to prepare and push around voluminous committee reports.

In this new situation the natural reaction of the decision makers — the politicians — would be to allocate public money directly to the local school with the governors — who are local people — and the Head of the school deciding what to do with it. They may want to spend their money on sending village children by bus to the town school. But it is much more likely that they would want to improve the village school. Any building that is necessary would mean work for local architects and builders. Also specialist part-time teachers might be employed. By spending the money locally the quality of education would change in the ways wanted by local people. This in turn would lead to the village becoming a more attractive place for families to choose to live in. The number of children would increase and so more money would be allocated to the school.

This kind of example can be found in every aspect of public service. The total effect, if decentralization came about, would be greater than the sum of all the parts added together because much more effective use would be made of the resources available locally than can be made by directives from the centre. The effect would be multiplied further in the longer term because the increasing decentralization of public services to the villages would lead to more self-sufficiency. Villages would become more attractive as places in which to live and this would lead to a growth of village shops and jobs.

The reduction of bureaucracy would mean that it would gradually become more and more attractive to set up village businesses. This would slow down or reverse the current trend towards bigger and bigger businesses and shops. A trend which has come about, amongst other reasons, because only large organizations can afford the head office manpower to cope with increasing red tape. Less bureaucracy would mean that it would be worthwhile to run small businesses.

Big businesses would find it increasingly difficult to have to deal with a wide range of attitudes from one locality to another. It is inconceivable that a small town in one part of the country would react the same way as another elsewhere. No two places want precisely the same things and businesses would have to decentralize their own organizations.

So the decentralization of public authority processes would tend to have the same effect on the private sector. The present trends towards dull uniformity would be replaced by more and more diversification. Local specialities of all kinds would evolve. Architectural styles and building techniques would become less standardized and more relevant to each locality. Public services would vary widely from area to area reflecting what people want. The trend towards sameness would be reversed.

How would the public spending money be distributed?

A centralist would argue that there has to be a bureaucracy at the centre to ensure that money is distributed in what he would see to be a fair and reasonable manner. In reality any method of distribution of resources from the centre must be arbitrary because the "formulae" invented by the bureaucrats cannot reflect what people and communities really want. In a democracy run on decentralized lines the distribution of resources would have to be done by those elected by the people to represent them. Political decisions on how the money should be spent would be more likely to reflect what people want — otherwise the future of the individual politicians would be in jeopardy.

With decentralization each local politician will have much more influence on what happens in his own area, and will be seen to be responsible for what happens by his electorate.

There is a hard truth underlying decentralization which many will find difficult to face up to. This is the inevitable shift of responsibility from the State to the individual. The quality of life will be de-standardized. For example, we will get a wider range of types and tastes of cheese in the shops, some water will be polluted, there will be more pot-holes in some roads, some buses will be less safe — and so on.

All these things are inevitable because there would not longer be an army of bureaucrats to "protect" us. But the overall quality and diversity of life will improve immeasurably compared with what would have happened if creeping centralization had been allowed to continue.

Introduction to Johan Galtung

TWO WAYS OF LIFE

The issues under consideration in this text are those of community, health, the nature of the connections between them and how those connections can be modified for the betterment of both. Johan Galtung moves us to another level of analysis — that of the individual quality of life within whatever community structure exists. He asks a very basic question — how to be happy.

There are many levels at which the analysis of health can be undertaken. Just how many depends on which definition of health and which theoretical perspective is used for the analysis. But it is helpful to consider at least five levels — individual, family, community, nation, and planet. Our focus in this text is community, but it is evident that all these levels interact, and the boundaries are clearly permeable. What Galtung does is to analyse the essential issue of quality in and of individual life. Starting with the premise that we have never been so rich but also so impoverished, he itemises some of the symptoms — the poor quality of the mass media, the marginalisation of spiritual issues, and the rising rate of mental illness. The causative factors he lists include ecological breakdown, individualism, education, conflict, and competition.

In short, he says, our problem is the Bourgeois Way of Life (BWL) — not bourgeois in the strict Marxist sense but in the older sense of being a burgher. This is a person who retreats inside the burgh to avoid the more unpleasant aspects of life; a process which has formed Western social structure.

But what we need now is not BWL but AWL — an Alternative Way of Life. The AWL can be seen as a contrast to the BWL; but hybridisation between the two has taken place, and the result is a ground plan for a more satisfying way of life.

There is a long tradition of approaching mental illness through a consideration of social and structural factors. Far less attention has been paid to mental health, and even less to mental health promotion. Yet it may well be the case that both mental illness and mental health stand in need of reconceptualisation.

Let me give two examples. Since the World Health Organisation defined health back in 1948 as a far more positive state than merely the absence of illness — something more related to the optimum functioning of a person — it has become a truism to say that health is much more than the elimination of disease. Different writers have attempted to clarify just how, in different terms. There is, however, a consensus that health is far more than the absence of symptoms of distress; it is a state which facilitates, in David Seedhouse's words, the achievement of potential. But so often this debate has been carried out in the context of physical health, and little time has been spent thinking through the implications for mental health.

What would be the characteristics of optimum mental health? Again, a great deal more than the absence of disease or distress. But what? Different cultural traditions have addressed this question, and the classical Hindu approach is to analyse the components of human consciousness as *Sat, Chit, Ananda* — being, awareness, and bliss. Bliss, however, is a hard word for some of us. Galtung offers happiness, and maybe in the analysis of community mental health the happiness of the individual is a good place to begin.

FURTHER READING

Morris Berman (1981) **The Reenchantment of the World**. Cornell Univ. Press.

Mike Money (1992) **The Shamanic Path to Mental Health Promotion**. In Trent, D. R. and Reed, C. *Promotion of Mental Health Vol. 2, 1992*. Avebury.

David Seedhouse (1986) **Health — The Foundation for Achievement**. Wiley.

World Health Organization (1988) **From Alma-Ata to the Year 2000**. WHO.

TWO WAYS OF LIFE

JOHAN GALTUNG

Contrasting the BWL (Bourgeois Way of Life) and AWL (Alternative Way of Life), Johan Galtung suggests that the meaning of our existence is to develop a capacity to be happy and spread some of it to our neighbours.

WITH WHOM YOU do what, how, when, where and why; that would be, more or less, a definition of a way of life. Without answers to these questions all exercises in the theory and practice of social change, become futile. For what is the purpose of even the most perfect structure if the lives lived inside that edifice are empty?

There have always been rich and wealthy people around and only a few of them have led lives that are real sources of inspiration to others. I am not thinking of the lofty ideals, of the highest levels of human development in terms of transpersonal union, sacred or secular, far beyond one's own little body, mind and soul. I am just thinking of one little but rather basic point: the capacity to be happy and spread some happiness, some basic sense of well-being, to others — at least to the nearest ones.

When the rich and wealthy did not exude happiness but even led miserable lives, like that recluse, the multi-billionaire Howard Hughes, there were always some explanations why liberation from the toil for survival did not liberate more positive human forces. One was the old religious one: that human beings are not good enough. Another that elites had already been destroyed in the struggle — but in that case their offspring should do better. Another, more socialist, was that the upper classes were condemned to spiritual and human misery anyhow, and that only the oppressed — the working classes, the non-whites, the tribals, the women — still had the human qualities that would make a difference. Given access to life in material dignity new man, *el hombre nuevo*, would arise. But socialist and social democratic changes took place, the welfare state came with precisely that material dignity (and is now probably on its way out) and new man/woman looked very much like the old one. An enormous increase in *quantity* of materially comfortable living did not seem to affect the *quality* of human life that much. Except in a negative sense: some basic worries had been engineered away. Example: Nordic people seem to have less money in the bank and to consume more gladly because they feel relatively well protected against the inescapable calamities of illness and old age, not to mention the two of them at the same time. This is less the case with North Americans than with North Europeans, one possible reason why the concern for money is so much out in the open (and often leads to so many rather unsavoury practices) on the other side of the Atlantic.

Nonetheless, a basic fact is that we have never been so rich, and yet so poor. Look at our mass media with its predigested, chopped-up material for the eyes and ears, an insult to the "masses" for whose consumption it is said to be produced and distributed. Look at the lack of spirituality of any kind except in small, marginalized groups. Look at all the indicators of disintegration, from mental disorders, alcoholism and other forms of drug addiction and suicide, via homicide, assault and robbery and rape and other forms of criminality, to the enormity of the violence in internal and external wars. It is very hard to sustain any hypothesis to the effect that human beings have somehow become better, that economic and social development have brought human development.

The socialist, and particularly the social democratic mistake seems obvious and has been pointed out very often: there was no basic critique of the Western social formation, only of the limited access. Contemporary green, alternative, even anarchist critique tries to go deeper into the roots of the social formation itself, hoping to identify factors that may have a bearing on the problem. The list is long, and would include such factors as:

Nature: *ecological breakdowns*, partly the cause and partly the effect of our lack of concern for nature, making co-existence, partnership, learning from nature more difficult. Breeding animals to kill them and eat them is a part of that syndrome.
Human: an intense *individualism*, bent at short-term maximization of individual utility combined with a *materialism* that sees the utility in material/somatic terms, as "satisfaction". It is assumed that others do the

same, that individualism and not collectivism is the rule, even inside the family, among friends, in the home, at school, at work. Solidarity is out!
Social: *careerism*, in order to get into the higher reaches of society, to get wealthy (economy), powerful (polity), famous (culture); above all to get the money needed to satisfy individual, material goals. That this leads to conflicts is obvious.
World: *competition, conflict, war,* each country trying to do at the world level what individuals do at the social level, maximizing national utility, defining that in economic, material terms as growth, capital accumulation and turnover, market shares, etc. That this leads to conflicts is obvious.

This is the description of a way of life and not only of social structures and processes. I have called that way of life: BWL: *Bourgeois Way of Life*, interpreting "bourgeois" not in the Marxist sense but rather historically, as the people living inside the *burg*, the *burghers*. They have four major characteristics:
Non-manual work: away from anything that has to do with direct contact with nature, leading to careerism.
Material comfort: dampening all the fluctuations of nature, creating distance to nature and hence easily leading to ecological breakdowns.
Privatism: withdrawal into family and peer groups, withdrawal into oneself as one's own social universe, engaged in bargains with others.
Security: trying to secure this existence against any kind of threat, at present seeing the nation state as the *burg* behind which security can be found provided the country is wealthy, strong and powerful.
The correspondence is obvious; they are taken out of the same social logic and social ethos. To break with BWL is in a very real sense to break with the Western social formation. As this is the formation within which we live, to live an alternative way of life, an AWL, is already to be a dissident, even to search for one is subversive activity, *if one has a choice*.
An AWL has some basic themes on which variations can be made. The main themes are, of course, to mix manual and non-manual work, to live closer to nature in a less artificial environment, to live more collectively in a setting of "mutual rights and obligations", and to generate more security in that setting, at a more direct, interpersonal level. The closeness to nature has to be sufficient to create more personal interest in avoiding ecological breakdowns simply by being more a part of the system, directly hit when something goes wrong. The collectivism has to be sufficient to generate a type of solidarity that makes one feel the

suffering of others sufficient to want to help. The general change in way of life would make careerism inside the present social formation look out of order, like an anachronism. Of course, one may play the role, even draw a salary, but skillfully avoid "top" positions (heads of ministries on the political or technical side, top manager of corporations, director of think tanks, ambassadorships etc.) letting one's body engage in ritual exercises within the system so as to leave the soul free to wander and wonder. The source of security would be near rather than remote and particularly not in pension funds subject to the ups and downs of the world money market and the fate of the nation state in which one happens to be born.

In this view of alternative ways of life there is a mix of two elements: a socio-political philosophy, *and* a personal choice, an existential resolve, to start here and now, not to wait till the coming of the revolution, or the crisis. In this ambiguity there are certain advantages for the "alternativists", and possibly for the society as a whole.

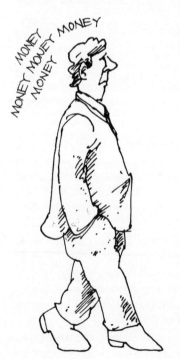

First, social experiments take place within the social formation, using its liberal potential, sometimes stretching it beyond the limits of tolerance. That many such experiments in ways of life (more healthy nutrition habits, more relaxed ways of relating to others, particularly to people "high up", more relaxed ways of dressing, etc.) have caught on, been accepted, is not to be doubted.

Second, exactly because a *choice* is needed there is a certain self-selection, meaning that those most motivated would be most likely to participate. Nobody is forced into an alternative way of life. By birth in the Western social formation one is launched into BWL, but with the possibility of opting out, at least to some extent, thanks to the level of liberalism found within that formation.

Third, a society is emerging due to this ambiguity with a mixture of BWL and AWL. Not necessarily a bad society. People can spin their life-lines through both life-styles and develop their own compromises. They can gamble on both horses, so to speak, maybe BWL for quantity (money, life expectancy) and AWL for quality (meaning, life experience). Society itself may be strengthened through this exercise in applied ecology: symbiotic diversity at work. Not only the individual who knows how to combine the two, but society becomes richer. The only ones to suffer are the purists, who want AWL to prevail totally and completely, into the deepest and innermost corners of society, and those who want BWL to keep its position of monopoly, except on the marginals, of course who by their very marginality prove the marginality of any AWL.

Why and for what reason do we need to exercise our brains to create a way of life? I think the religious answer is right: it must be for human development, in harmony with nature. It cannot be social development or world development; they must be means rather than ends, conditions rather than the consequences of our activities. Actually, this is precisely what is so troublesome about such Western political ideologies as liberalism (blue), marxism (red) and anarchism (green): all these blue-prints for perfect social structures tend to take on value in their own right as if the whole goal of life is to create the social and world edifice.

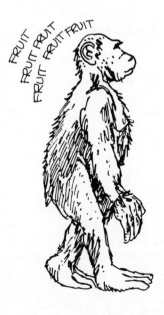

LET ME BE CONCRETE. When one is young and trained in BWL one of the first things to learn is "postponement of gratification". *First* you have to do this, *then* comes the time for enjoyment. The dessert is in the end, if at all. The young human being is given some years of irresponsible enjoyment as childhood; then comes Education. Education is organized as a chain of schools, first primary, then secondary, then tertiary. All the time the message is the same: first you must have your exam 1, 2, 3 etc., then Life starts. But after all those exams comes Work which is also or-ganized as a staircase with levels, 1, 2, 3, get your promotions then Life starts.

Quite soon the last phase comes, Retirement. Presumably that is when Life really starts, towards the end, when Death is approaching.

A cruel system. I am not even sure if it is an effective way of squeezing work out of people. Against this serial arrangement of Life in four phases, CEWR (using the initials of the four phases) I would strongly argue in favour of a more relaxed, more random model. Take a year or two of childhood, then some work, then some education, then a little retirement, then some work again, some childhood, some education. Construct your own life series, mix the elements. It will probably not be good for your individual "career" in the BWL-dominated society. But it may be very good for your own inner growth, with a lot of experience, letting the parts play together into patterns for your own construction, making you yourself and others less obviously predictable because the life series are so painfully similar.

Very concretely: *start living now*. This is not an argument against a good dose of education, but an argument against continuous, consecutive schooling, letting the schools come in the way of other forms of living. For this flexibility is needed, even at the individual and social levels. Generally that flexibility has to be created. In my own case I have found freelancing to be one answer. In economic terms it has the advantage of being paid for what one does, the market satisfaction of matching supply and demand, which I do not scorn. One is not paid a salary regardless of how one performs, for instance as a professor. The disadvantage is also clear: there is not only predictability but also security in that regular pay-slip.

There is a social counterpart to this postponement of gratification idea: postponement till after the liberation/revolution. A friend of mine (ex-marxist) once said, recommending very strongly the movie "From Mao to Mozart": that is the kind of life one should have after the revolution! Himself an accomplished amateur musician he felt this was Life, exploring the delights of sublime music, on string instruments. I agree, this is the kind of thing people should do, those who want to do so. Others might be concerned with the intricacies of theology/ philosophy; for instance, the deeper problems of Buddhist thought or human capacity for self-improvement. Still others might prefer math-ematics: I remember myself as a student of mathematics, before the final exam, agreeing that some differential equations (great fun to solve, actually) could be enjoyed at the old age home, not *now*. Now is exam. Still others would prefer to create with their hands, objects, artefacts, art.

It is as if society, like individuals, needs a diploma before enjoyment can start, a clean bill of health, or whatever. A certificate of revolutionary excellence. To use a brutal example: it becomes like all these people I have met in my life who not only are dishonest but (a) know they are dishonest in the sense of concealing their true views and (b) consider this very smart — better be a conformist on the surface in order not to make trouble for yourself; and then, when you are through with Education, or when you are well launched in Work, *then* comes the great exercise of honesty to prove yourself and shock the world. Chances are that day never comes, the honesty was killed in the process. Moral: honesty, like life, starts here and now, but to be honest does not mean to be inconsiderate.

Meaning and happiness for oneself and one's surroundings have to be one's own creation. They are not incompatible with worries about security; but there is a limit. Worries about survival, individually or collectively, from starvation or nuclear war; worries about survival, individually or collectively, from starvation or nuclear war; worries about basic needs due to fluctuations in market conditions; worries about basic freedoms because of mounting repression, all of these cannot but interfere with the search for meaning and happiness. And yet, the struggle for a better society and a better world should come in addition to the struggle for meaning and happiness, not prior to them, as a pre-condition.

But, one may object, could not meaning and happiness be found, even created, exactly in the struggle to set the society and world right? No. This is the old problem so brilliantly analyzed by Koestler in *The Yogi and the Commissar*. The Commissar may succeed in making an edifice, but it is unfit for the Yogi to live in. The Yogi may come very far in human growth, but at the expense of withdrawing from society, creating his own little hermitage, ultimately only with one inhabitant, himself. The Commissar does not develop the faculties for inner growth in his political work and the yogi does not develop the capacity to change the social order. Obviously the answer is some kind of both-and, which is the reason for recommending parallel activity. To the question "Where shall we start, changing ourselves or changing the world", the answer is both simultaneously.

So, *what* does one do, *how*, *where* and *when*? Maybe we have much to learn from the monastic orders. The best ones were and are micro societies (except for not being biologically reproductive given the norms of celibacy), combining manual and non-manual work. Time is split between what is necessary for survival, well-being and security and what is deemed sufficient, by that order, for inner human growth. Monasteries are compromises between the Commissar, who only goes in for the former, and the Yogi, only going for the latter. One is amazed by their capacity to survive, not unchanged, but basically unmolested by the running of history. Of course, longevity is not an end in itself, but it is an indicator of some basic adequacy. Just think of how they matched scenic beauty with architectural and artistic aestheticism! Take the Ajanta caves in Maharashtra state in India, Buddhist refuges in an increasingly hostile environment!

And yet we probably do not want to live in monasteries, partly because we do not believe in celibacy, partly because we may not believe in that much isolation. So, relax the rules a little, or much. Make it easier to join and leave. Build on the element of self-reliance and the focus on human growth and the idea that time for essentials is *now*, not after the world has been set straight and right — meaning never. Create a commune, a neighbourhood, a sense of community, even spread out in space; using the excellent telecommunication facilities of our age, even quite inexpensive at non-peak hours. Create networks, flexible, avoid heavy centralization, associate across all kinds of borders, and there is even an answer to the *with whom* problem. Potentially with anybody who is pulling somehow in the same general direction. And they are very numerous, today, indeed. More than numerous enough to get started *now. Anywhere.* And both with inner growth and outer change.

Johan Galtung is Professor of Peace Studies at the Universities of Witten-Heidecke and Hawaii. He is one of the most renowned peace researchers of our times.

Published in *Resurgence* No. 111, July/August 1985.

Introduction to Michael Phillips and Greta Alexander

A NEW WAY TO DO BUSINESS

Economics matters; and any world-view that pretends it doesn't soon runs out of cash. Economics matters to communities, because if a community's economic structure allows all its cash be syphoned off, you end up with an impoverished community and quite soon no community at all. This lesson has been learned the hard way by many communities in both Europe and the Third World, who have been victims of well-intentioned but socially destructive development. It may sound materialistic, but just as one of the best predictors of how healthy an elderly person will be is how much money he or she has, so quantity of cash is quite a good predictor of community health.

But let me make two caveats. The first is that cash may be a necessary condition for community health; but it's not sufficient. There's a saying, "If you want to know what God thinks of money, look at the people s/he gives it to." And as Galtung illustrated in the previous article with his example of Howard Hughes, money does not necessarily bring happiness. The second caveat is that there is more than one way of conceptualizing cash, and more than one way of keeping count. Credit Unions, cooperatives, community banks and local currencies may all have their part to play in the development of healthy communities.

So too does business, which generates and circulates wealth. Current centralist consumerist economics means that most of us are engaged in what William Morris called useless toil, rather than in useful work; and that money spent on a pair of trousers in Liverpool on Tuesday is in a Swiss bank by the following night. Both processes impoverish communities; both stem from a particular view of economics and business.

But Phillips and Alexander show us that there is another way to run a business. They call it the Briarpatch Network; named after the briarpatch in which Brer Rabbit hid from predators. The American Briarpatch network of 600 businesses is rooted in honesty and service to the community. Members only consider business ventures that conserve natural resources, entail having fun, and allow their owners to have simple lifestyles. More unusually, they make their bookkeeping records and financial transactions public. Clients can see how much profit was made from their work — if it was excessive, they can negotiate a better price next time.

Briars also network together to help one another with business problems, and are committed to helping people with the same ideals to get started. And before they are written off as unpractical idealists, while the national United States statistics for businesses going broke in their first three years is 80%, the figure for the Briars is 5%. The Briarpatch network is a model for those who would start or revitalise community businesses. And communities need them; in the transition to a sustainable society development must start from the sustainable community. Local businesses play a key role in such sustainability. They ensure local wealth, provide employment for the young, and meaningful, satisfying work in and for the community. When based at home, they are less likely to exploit or pollute their neighbours. And their significance for happiness and health cannot be overestimated.

FURTHER READING

Guy Dauncey (1988) **After the Crash — The Emergence of the Rainbow Economy**. Green Print.

Paul Ekins (1986) **The Living Economy**. Routledge & Kegan Paul.

James Robertson (1989) **Future Wealth: A New Economics for the 21st Century**. Cassell.

A NEW WAY
TO DO BUSINESS

MICHAEL PHILLIPS & GRETA ALEXANDER

**Social concerns and business have a history of conflict.
Marxism was proposed as a way to eliminate conflict by
placing ownership with the State. The Co-op movement of the
nineteenth century was another approach, placing ownership
in the hands of suppliers or consumers of the business.
Employee ownership is still another approach, with the
Mondragon group in Basque Spain as a good example. An
alternative approach successful in the United States is based
on the assumption that business and social concerns are not
in basic conflict. This approach is most highly developed in
the San Francisco Bay Area where 600 businesses, calling
themselves the Briarpatch, have been participating in a
network for eight years.**

T HIS GROUP OF businesses is called the Briarpatch Network
and its members are called Briars. The Network is an informal
association of people and businesses who share common values
and are untraditional in a few ways but similar to your own neighbourhood businesses in others.

The Briarpatch Network differs from more traditional associations
because the Network seldom has meetings and officers; it usually has
parties, classes in how to improve business practices and has a group of
advisors (financial, legal and accounting) to help members of the
Network. The Network invariably has one or two co-ordinators. They
help put businesses with common problems or questions in contact with
each other and publish a directory of members.

In San Francisco, the co-ordinator of the Network is Shali Parsons, who spends a typical day answering a few phone calls from Briars... one call might be about writing a partnership agreement. The caller would be referred to a book on do-it-yourself partnerships published by Nolo Press, another Briarpatch member that publishes self-help legal books. A second call might be from a small neighbourhood grocery store wanting advice on whether or not to expand to an adjacent vacant space. Shali would arrange for a visit to the store by several Briarpatch financial advisors. For this range of services, Briarpatch members make voluntary contributions of money, or barter services, every six months. The fees and donations support the co-ordinator on a part-time basis and pay for the parties and periodic mailings to members.

Networks already exist in Northern California and the area around Eugene, Oregon. A recent one started in 1981 in Seattle, Washington, calling itself the Potlatch Network. "Potlatch" is the name of the Northwest Indian ritual of sharing food and wealth.

The word "Briarpatch" is derived from the African tales of Uncle Remus, in which the hero, Brer Rabbit, leads a happy, safe life in the thicket of thorns called a briarpatch. The gentle rabbit is protected from predators by its humble and seemingly inhospitable home. Briar business people feel that attention to keeping their lives simple and their businesses open and honest protects them from the attention and problems of the larger society.

The Briar values of honesty and service to the community can be found in many traditional businesses in small towns and neighbourhoods everywhere. In big cities they are just beginning to find each other and form networks to provide support for their shared values.

The 600 Briarpatch businesses in the San Francisco Bay Area include nearly every kind of business from a high fashion clothing designer (Kaisek Wong), to a massage-table manufacturer (Living Earth Products); it includes lawyers, book publishers, magazines, artists, grocery stores and computer companies.

Mixed in the assortment of members is a sheep ranch that has thousands of sheep (Bell Ranch), an elegant $2 million restaurant and a unique and highly respected school. There is a special library of medical information available to the public (Planetree), many holistic medical practitioners, clinics and schools. A Japanese acupuncturist, an Irish bar (Finnegan's Wake), a Mexican weaving company, an Asian Theatre troupe, a Tea Ceremony school and an immigration lawyer. Almost any service or product you could want is available in the San Francisco

Briarpatch, plus dozens of fascinating businesses that are completely new ideas.

The outwardly visible characteristics of the people who run Briarpatch businesses is that most are under forty-five years old, there is a high proportion of women owners, and in talking to Briars you find their values have been heavily influenced by the ideas and experiences of the social/political/environmental upheaval which occurred in the United States during the late 1960s and 1970s... the Vietnam War/Hippies/Ecology/Civil Rights era. Today they are very successful entrepreneurs running their businesses in a way that reflects the new social visions of ecology and social justice. What are these values and how are they reflected in the 600 Briarpatch businesses?

The first is love of their business. Business is a way to serve others. This separates them from the values of many small businesses who are working to make money. Not the Briars. Because of their environmental values, they only engage in businesses that preserve resources, that allow the owners to seek simple lifestyles and to have fun in their work. They definitely are not in business to take a lot of money. One of the heroes of the Briarpatch is Stewart Brand, publisher of the *Whole Earth Catalogue*. This enormously successful book had a net profit of over $1.25 million. Stewart created a board of directors to give the money away to worthwhile environmental and political-action causes relevant to the issues discussed in the *Whole Earth Catalogue*. Today, Stewart publishes the *Co-Evolution Quarterly* (in Sausalito, California), a Briarpatch magazine containing articles about current leading-edge ecological issues. Another Briar is Kaisek Wong, the high fashion clothing designer, who loves the fashion business but hates to employ and supervise people. Kaisek and his mother sew all the clothes he designs; when you buy one of his dresses, you really have an original. Even though demand is great and the prices customers are willing to pay continues to rise (now over $2,000 per dress), Kaisek will not hire anyone else to sew for him. He doesn't believe in expansion for its own sake. The same is true of George DeWoody whose "Image Development" graphic design firm in San Francisco was so successful that its business doubled every year. When he reached five employees, George said, "That's enough. I'm a graphic designer, I want to design; not supervise other designers. No more employees. From now on we take only work that we want to do, work that is challenging and fun." That was in 1979. Today, "Image Development" is one of the most sought-after graphic designers in the western United States and still has a total of five employees.

The second value that Briarpatch businesses have in common that reflects their social values and distinguishes them from more traditional businesses is that their book-keeping records are open and financial transactions are public. In any Briarpatch business you can ask to see the financial statements, ask how much rent is paid for the space and what they pay for supplies... you will be given a clear, understandable answer and explanation. Many Briar businesses publish their financial statements; the *CoEvolution Quarterly* does and so does *Common Ground* (a listing of Religious/New Age/Transformational organizations) and *The People's Yellow Pages* (a listing of social service agencies). *CoEvolution* once found that by publishing their printing expenses resulted in printers all over the United States offering lower bids for printing.

Most Briarpatch businesses have had similar experiences. Honest people running open businesses results in better management, more community support and an opportunity for friends and family to actively participate in the business.

One wonderful example of open books is Sven Olmstead of Stockholm, Sweden, a Briar who runs a successful building contracting business. Sven builds homes, offices and factories for a fixed contract price and lets his customers see his financial statements. Sven explains the results: "When clients see that I have lost money on a project, the client is very appreciative of the hard work and excess effort my company made to do a good job for them; these clients always come back to me for their next job. When I make a large profit it is visible and the clients also come back, insisting that I offer them low bids — after all, I 'made lots of money on the last job I did for them.' "

Being open with financial information is like having an open kitchen in a fine restaurant... it is a reflection of the pride that the chef has in her/his cooking. In an ordinary restaurant when patrons ask to see the kitchen, they are often told, "We are busy right now... our insurance doesn't permit people in the kitchen. Of course, it is reasonable to assume that such a restaurant has a dirty kitchen and uses frozen food in microwave ovens. Similarly, the open books of the Briarpatch businesses are a sign of pride, a willingness to learn and a high degree of honesty is directed at providing quality service to their customers.

A third quality Briars have in common is their generosity with other people outside the Network. As an example, The Down Depot which cleans down sleeping-bags, parkas and jackets has helped other Briar outdoor rental businesses to clean their used sleeping-bags at a low price and on a rush basis; they have also trained dozens of people who wanted to start down cleaning stores in other parts of the United States. The same is true for Toy-Go-Round (Albany, California), which sells used toys. Children who bring their used toys to Toy-Go-Round receive 50% of the sale price when their item is sold. The owners often help community charities sell toys their members bring in. They have trained many people to run similar stores in other parts of the country. They also advise parents who inquire which toys are safest and last longest.

The most surprising fact about the Briarpatch way of doing business is their extraordinary success and survival rate. In the United States the average failure rate is 80% in the first three years of business... Briars experience less than 5% in three years.

The Briarpatch way of doing business can be found everywhere. It is growing in cities and metropolitan areas as people find each other and form networks. Briarpatch Networks spread very much like plants; the seeds have to be carried to a new area where they can grow in fertile soil. Most of the networks that were started after San Francisco, were started by Briars who had moved from The Bay Area. They felt lonely without other people to share the excitement of business and their concerns about social issues so these people got together and formed new networks.

Because the Briarpatch way of doing business has such a successful record of helping people run their business, Briarpatch Networks will spread ultimately to many areas where there are clusters of business which also value service, quality, openness and sharing. Experience so far indicates that it takes a minimum of twenty businesses to get a network started and seventy to keep it going.

The Briar way of doing business will also spread because people come from all over the world to look at the new types of business that have started in the Bay Area Network. Briars offer help and encourage people to start similar businesses everywhere. The openness and success of the Briars in doing business based on honesty and sharing is contagious. Many of the new enterprises are started in other areas with financial statements open to the public and business designed to be deliberately small scale.

Probably the most important lesson that the Briarpatch has to teach is its view of the future. The Briarpatch view is that the future will not be better if it is based solely on technology. While many view the future as a time when people will fly around on platforms, live in outer space, and have robots to serve them... Briars believe that the future will not even exist unless people change their interpersonal relations. Briars practice their view that we will only survive if we learn to share with each other, act openly, and strive for simpler lives that preserve scarce resources and serve others. Technology does not hold any hope for the future if people don't learn to behave differently. And since business is such a fundamental part of each person's life... it is the source of food, clothing, housing and communications and transportation... that business must reflect new personal values. One Briarpatch business that is a good example of this is the Owner Builder Centre. It is a school that has been growing very rapidly, getting more and more students each year. It teaches people how to build their own houses and how to remodel houses they live in. The classes are taught by teachers with many years of practical experience who actually work with the students on their own houses and remodelling projects. It is cooperation on a very high level with access to the latest solar and electronic technology.

The Briarpatch is an exciting and wonderful development but not many people know about it. The reason is that Briars do not believe in proselitizing. They strongly believe in their own values but they don't try to convince or convert other people. They look for other people who share the same values and they support each other. This article is written to encourage other people to help each other and share the Briarpatch optimism. Please don't try to write or phone the Briarpatch Network; they don't have descriptive material to mail out and the co-ordinator is very happy working part-time. He doesn't want phone calls from people who are curious.

Start your own Briarpatch with a party and invite other business people who share your values.

Michael Phillips is the founder of the Briarpatch Network and author of several books including **Seven Laws of Money***. Greta Alexander ran a successful business for many years designing, creating and marketing fine handmade jewellery. At the time of writing she was a marketing representative for a major corporation.*

Published in *Resurgence* No. 98, May/June 1983.

Introduction to A.T. Ariyaratne

NO POVERTY SOCIETY

A.T. Ariyaratne writes from thirty years of experience in Sri Lanka's Sarvodaya Shramadana movement, whose name means "awakening of all through mutual sharing".

Ariyaratne's article continues the economic theme. Reflecting a perspective familiar from the work of E.F. Schumacher, he itemises some of the principles through which the development of a healthy human society can be attained.

Profoundly decentralist in orientation, he argues that change will come from the poor rather than the rich. The rich are insulated from the severest symptoms of social and economic breakdown; they can choose to involve themselves in some project or enterprise, but as Peter Nabokov has observed, good-hearted environmentalists can always go home when it gets tiresome. But, like the poor, "Inhabitory peoples will fight for their lives like they've been jumped in an alley..."

Very large organisations offer little hope of real change, partly for the reasons discussed by Cooper. At best they can be used as sources of funding and information.

So how do communities conform more to an equitable and sustainable way of life? Ariyaratne stresses five elements:

- Keeping faith with traditional values
- Using appropriate technology to increase community participation in those processes which meet community need
- Assisting community organisations to attain full legal status
- Networking around and through the formal administrative processes to affect decision-making
- Forming supportive relationships with other, similar organisations.

The Sarvodaya movement did not begin with structured theory such as this — it was evolved from a process of active involvement which fell into three stages. The first phase of the movement focused on working in villages where poor and marginalised groups required assistance; a process which ultimately involved over 350,000 people working in hundreds of camps all over the country, and which entailed projects such as building roads and schools, constructing wells and toilets, and helping people to develop the skills required for constructive, collaborative work.

The second phase was explicit community development, in which all aspects of integrated village development were carried out by villagers themselves with the assistance of movement members. This took place in more than a thousand villages all over Sri Lanka. The third phase was global; an ongoing process of working for partnership with all other people: every individual, family, village and urban community.

Ariyaratne advocates a holistic approach to community development; and emphasises the actual and potential role of technology in either magnifying or reversing those processes which make for material poverty. For example, the development of microelectronics will soon remove the advantages of cheap skilled labour from third world markets. So countries affected by changes like this will be forced to seek sustainable economies. The World Bank model of development is something to be rejected, he feels, if only because the interest on the sort of capital investment necessary to enable a country like Sri Lanka to compete with the West on equal terms would result in crippling debt. Rather than following this top-down model of development, grassroots action of the sort outlined by Schumacher is far more likely to result in real global change to a dynamic world culture.

There are many fascinating elements in Ariyaratne's account. But the one that intrigues me the most, perhaps, is the extent to which his model of community development through education and grassroots economics is transferrable to contexts such as our own, where similar problems of poverty and marginalisation contribute substantially to ill-health, and still await resolution.

FURTHER READING

Ivan Illich (1980) **Towards a History of Needs**. Bantam.

E.F. Schumacher (1974) **Small is Beautiful**. Abacus.

NO POVERTY SOCIETY

A. T. ARIYARATNE

A. T. Ariyaratne is unique among men involved in rural development by introducing the gift of human labour as the main tool of the upliftment of the poor. He has nurtured the spirit and the energy of the people to work for the good of their communities.

I AM GRATEFUL TO the Schumacher Society for this opportunity given to me to deliver a Schumacher Lecture this year. My very special thanks should go to my dear friend, Satish Kumar, who invited me to perform this task in spite of his knowledge about the inadequacy of my academic achievements compared to the high standards already set by the earlier speakers of this lecture series who were people of great intellectual attainment and philosophical eminence. Further I am honoured, and in a sense inspired, by the presence of George McRobie, the life-long friend and co-worker of Dr Schumacher, who helped him show to the world that small was possible. I consider George not only a friend very close to my heart, but a teacher who guided me in many ways to do the small and beautiful things we are doing back home in Sri Lanka.

Before I come to the subject I have chosen to speak to you about this evening, namely, "Blazing a Path for the World's Poor and the Powerless — Towards a No-Poverty Society", I think it is appropriate that I make some remarks about my association with the late Dr E. F. Schumacher.

I was born and bred in a village in Sri Lanka. As a youth, the more I came in contact with what is now generally known as modern urban life, the more I withdrew almost intuitively back into my rural society with its lively Buddhist cultural values. I increasingly believed that life can be meaningful and human fulfilment can be achieved only in small organized communities where social, political and economic life is guided by spiritual, moral and cultural values. Naturally this urge led me to India several times in the late fifties and early sixties to witness how Acharya Vinoba Bhave and Shri Jayaprakash Narayan were translating the Gandhian ideals into concrete action through the Bhoodan-Gramdan Movement.

It was during this period that I had the good fortune to meet briefly Dr Schumacher both at the Gandhian Institute of Studies in Varanasi and the Gandhi Peace Foundation in New Delhi. But it was in the early seventies when he visited our work in Sri Lanka that we became intimate friends. Subsequently I visited his home twice with my brother who was living in England at that time.

In February 1976, TOOL — an Appropriate Technology Organization in the Netherlands, which was headed by another friend of mine, Ton de Wilde (who is presently the Executive Director of Appropriate Technology International in Washington), organized an international conference in Nijmegen. Dr Schumacher was invited to deliver the keynote address and I was asked to make the first response after his speech. It so happened that Dr Schumacher's flight from London was delayed and he couldn't make it in time for the opening address. I remember just five minutes before the congress opened he telephoned the President of the Congress, talked to him first, and then I was called to the telephone. In his inimitable voice he said, "It is you who will give the keynote and I will come and respond to what you say." My most vehement protests didn't work and the next minute I was speaking on a subject I hardly knew. A couple of hours later he was there, saw the video and responded to my remarks in such a manner that his thoughts on technology and development became an integral part of the *Sarvodaya Shramadana* Movement and my own thinking from that day.

I met him last in Vienna at the International Voluntary Service Conference a few months before his untimely demise. He was telling me about declaring the following year a "year of moratorium" from his work. As you and I now know he never did that. He couldn't do that. The demands from the world and the urgency within him to deliver his message to humanity was such that he passed away while on his mission. Now it is our task to pick up from where he left and continue the good work.

I believe that I can honour his name best by not referring to his epoch-making book *Small is Beautiful* and the other works that followed, but by sharing with you our experience in trying to realize some of his ideas in practice.

I WILL REFER only to one idea he expressed in an address he delivered under the title "A Metaphysical Basis for Decentralization".

"... I would suggest that possibilities for any real change, not in the taking but in the doing, can only come from small groups of people. In a sense we don't really need a theory of decentralization. The dinosaurs will collapse under their own weight. Innovating minorities are always small and are ipso facto decentralized. If any one of us still expects any real help from big powerful organizations, I suggest he is wasting his time. These organizations are big and powerful precisely because they are not, in this sense, innovating. So the best thing to do is to forget them, or even better, if you are clever enough, to use them as milch cows."

The *Sarvodaya Shramadana* Movement, from whose twenty-six year old experience I am speaking to you, is one such innovative effort by small groups of people living in over 7,000 rural communities in Sri Lanka. *Sarvodaya Shramadana* means Awakening of All through Mutual Sharing.

In our work we have come across four categories of people according to the life-styles they value. Firstly, those who are affluent and powerful and believe wealth and power to be the end purpose of life; secondly, those who aspire to achieve wealth and power in the belief that that is the way to a fuller life; thirdly, those who have achieved these but are still unhappy and looking for alternative modes of simpler living; and fourthly those who are poor and powerless but are quite satisfied if they are able to attain a No-Poverty Society in which they can live as free human beings within their cultural milieu.

The *Sarvodaya Shramadana* is a movement of the poor, by the poor for the Awakening of All, not excluding the awakening of the people belonging to the above-mentioned first three categories. We commence our work with the most deprived in our societies and totally depend on their leadership to initiate the processes that will lead to a post-modern society. As the well-known Gandhian scholar, the late Prof. Sugatha Das Gupta mentioned, our effort is not to build an alternative society but to proceed from the old society, that is from where we are, to a post-modern society which we believe is neither sustainable nor possible for all people in the world to attain.

The main tasks of the Movement as experienced during the last twenty-six years are as follows:

- Assist communities to re-affirm their faith in their traditional value systems as far as their relevance to their present-day realities of life are concerned;
- Strengthen their community participatory systems with appropriate technological skills enabling them to plan out and implement their own felt-need-satisfaction programmes;
- Assist community organizations to get incorporated as legal entities, thus enabling them to get the maximum benefits in the realization of their human rights in the economic and political life of the nation;
- Organize lateral networks of their own independent units at different levels of the administrative system of the country, enabling them to exert an influence on the decision-making processes by concrete examples; and
- Establish fraternal relationships with organizations and movements with similar objectives for mutual support.

We believe that these processes of self-development, thus promoted at the level of the individual, the family, the rural and urban communities the world over, will evolve themselves into a global movement so decisive that the present monocultural suicidal trend in our world can be radically changed.

I do not think that the present giant transnational organizations, be they political, industrial, commercial, monetary, technological or any other, can be made to act on the realization that a close relationship exists between the way their structures function and the increase in poverty, crimes, armed conflicts, wars, ecological destruction and cultural degeneration and so on going on in our societies. All these organizations seem to be controlled mostly by the first category of people I mentioned. Therefore, there is nothing significant that could be achieved, as Dr Schumacher rightly said, by appealing to them or placing before them facts and figures which we sometimes think they are unaware of. They know all that much better than we do. They simply have become the prisoners of what the present systems have created in the form of institutionalizing the baser instincts of man such as greed and ill will. When the inherent contradictions in these systems begin to hurt them seriously, only then will they think of the massive suffering that other human beings in the world are going through today. If this painful experience does not come too late for them, basic groups such as *Sarvodaya* may still be able to help them to join hands with the rest of humanity to build a more just, sustainable and peaceful society. If the realization comes too late, then we have to allow them to face themselves the consequences of universal laws of cause and effect.

What about the second and third categories of people, namely, those who aspire for affluence and have not yet fulfilled their desires, and those who are already affluent but are dissatisfied with what this has to offer by way of happiness? As far as the *Sarvodaya* Movement is concerned we try to assist them to change their world view and life-styles and, if they are prepared to make the sacrifice, to join hands with us to build a no-poverty-society.

So the choice before the world, and the poor in particular, is very clear. The task of building the new society, the post-modern society, is clearly the responsibility of the people who are poor and powerless and yet who have the intelligence and insight to realize the barrenness of a consumer-oriented mass-production violent society. The poor and the powerless, paradoxically enough, are the least confused and perplexed.

THE *SARVODAYA SHRAMADANA* effort in Sri Lanka did not begin with a ready-made theory which we had only to practise. It was a long arduous journey which we travelled, and still are travelling, making as intelligent responses as we possibly could to the challenges we faced as we went along.

Firstly, as young teachers and students we wanted to broaden our learning experience by going into the villages where our economically poor, socially depressed, and politically ostracized brothers and sisters lived. We combined our learning experience with a service component where we attempted to help improve their living conditions by sharing our labour and other resources we could find. I remember that there were over 200 communities at that time who were considered to be "backward communities" owing to the so-called "low" castes to which they were born. This was our first area of "study-service".

I also remember very vividly how these communities were objects of sociological study for some Western-educated Sri Lankan scholars who wrote books and theses after careful analysis of their caste origins and other matters such as inter-relationships, *but never cared to help these people to control their own destiny*. As young people we went to these academics for guidance and assistance to help these people lift up themselves by their own efforts. These academics asked us to approach them through the proper channels, namely through the heads of the Education Ministry. The bureaucracies of the educational authorities were also closed to us at that time as we were taking education away from the classroom, text-books and examinations to the "prohibited" area of the real life of the people.

The Study component of our programme was, and is, not for academic purposes. It is to help awaken our inner selves to the fullest potential in this life. Whatever knowledge we gain in the process is incidental and it helps us to be wiser in life. Such inner awakening takes place only through real life experience.

During this first phase of the Movement we managed to interest over 350,000 people, mostly youths, to participate in hundreds of *Shramadana* (mutual sharing of labour) camps in all parts of the country where people of diverse ethnic, religious and racial composition lived. We realized that *Shramadana* was an excellent means to help people to realize respect for all life, engage in compassionate actions, learn to discover the joy of service to fellow beings and develop an attitude of mind where gains and losses are faced with equanimity. Of course, the other positive benefits such as leadership development, building psychological bridges among people and numerous physical activities such as building roads, school-buildings, community halls, wells, toilets and so on were no less important.

During this ten-year period the Movement did not receive any local or foreign funding except some random assistance mainly from villagers themselves. Even today the main investment of the Movement is labour and services given free to *Sarvodaya* programmes by thousands of people.

THE SECOND PHASE of the Movement was a community development programme. We began with a hundred selected villages. All aspects of integrated village development were carried out by village people themselves and the Movement came in with additional volunteers, training components and whatever other material inputs it could find from outside. It is at this stage: that is, nearly fourteen years after the inception of the Movement, that some foreign developmental organiza-tions such as OXFAM (UK) came in to support us. Our principal input, however, was the resources of the people themselves and the effort put in by the willing hands from outside the village. By the end of 1972 we were working in well over 1,000 villages in our country.

The Third Phase of the Movement started around this time when we came to realize by practical experience that what was necessary was a total change in our understanding of development and the strategies and methodologies we were using, not only within the *Sarvodaya* Movement but also in other governmental and global approaches. We also realized that during our long period of struggle and interactions with both local and foreign development thinkers, practitioners, administrators and our partners that the path to a more just and peaceful life for our people, whether they are in Asia, Africa, Latin America, Europe, North America or any other place should be through an awakening process taking place in thousands of groups all over the globe. Together we should awaken at the level of the individual person, the family, the village and the urban community. Then and only then nations and the world as a whole would awaken.

This awakening should be total, integrating within it the spiritual, moral, cultural, social, economic and political life of man and society.

Sarvodaya is not offering a mono-cultural formula for all the ills in the world. On the other hand, by sheer hard work it has released an integrated series of processes in the above manner in over 7,000 village communities out of 23,000 in Sri Lanka involving the lives of over two and a half million people. In each village a programme based on self-reliance, community participation and a simple plan, decided upon by the people themselves, is implemented. From pre-school children, through school-going children, youths, mothers, farmers and other adults activities are planned and implemented. A village level *Sarvodaya Shramadana* Society is organized in due course and legally registered with the government. These societies then have opportunities to engage themselves in economic activities which benefit the village people. Also the power of the people as a whole for collective action is strengthened in the processes of working together in a variety of fields that affect their lives.

The village in its basic needs satisfaction programme needs a variety of trained people; pre-school workers, health-care workers, nutrition workers, community-shop keepers, savings-credit organizers, rural technical service workers, agriculture promoters and so on. These workers are trained at local, district and national level centres. There are about 360 such training centres where around 2,400 young people are given residential training at any one time. The headquarters of the Movement and several of the larger district centres cater to the needs of national, as well as the international, needs of the Movement. Most of the assistance the Movement receives is channelled into training of workers and strengthening of village level societies.

There are over 200 foreign students at any one time working and learning in *Sarvodaya* projects around the country, while 46 *Sarvodaya* youths are working in other developing countries in Asia and Africa in similar activities directly, sponsored by the *Sarvodaya Shramadana* International, or in co-operation with other fraternal organizations.

Sarvodaya has established close working relationships with several similar organizations around the world for experience exchange and for mutual support. There are several international non-governmental organizations supporting the Movement in various ways. There are also several intergovernmental organizations and three governmental organizations co-operating with *Sarvodaya* projects and programmes without infringing on our freedom. This is briefly the history and the present status of the *Sarvodaya Shramadana* Movement of Sri Lanka.

SARVODAYA WAS DEEPLY influenced by the teachings of the Buddha. We always considered the thought of the "Well-being of All" to be central to our work. Therefore from the inception of the Movement we rejected narrow sectarianism and worked *with* and *for* all, irrespective of their ethnic, religious or racial background. We were careful not to confine the participation in our Movement only to Buddhists or limit its services exclusively for Buddhist communities. From the beginning non-Buddhists participated in our work as equals and about thirty percent of the villages we are working in at present are inhabited mostly by people who are Hindus, Muslims or Christians. I mention this fact because there are deliberate and mischievous attempts made by some armchair critics to convey a false view of our religious stand.

Writing a foreword to his classical work on the Mediaeval Sinhalese Art in 1908 Dr Ananda K. Coomaraswamy says:

> "What are the conditions necessary to the existence of a worthy art? Let us first enquire what conditions forbid its existence in the modern West. They may be summed up in the words commercialism and irreligion."

He continues later in the same foreword:

> "... A society which sees wealth in things rather than in men, is ultimately doomed. It appears, therefore, that it is absolutely essential that mechanical production in the future be not abandoned, but controlled in the real interests of humanity. If this appears to be impossible, as I am unwilling to believe, it must be admitted that civilization is not much better than a failure; for it is not much good

being more ingenious than our forefathers if we cannot be either happier or better."

In our present affluent societies, not only in art but in every department of life, irreligion and commercialism play the dominant roles. We need a dynamic spiritual revival in religion and a radical replacement of commercialism. I do not have a formula to place before you as to how to achieve this. But I have no doubt that the way for a happier and better life for mankind lies in a holistic approach to life and society where spiritual and material development take place harmoniously. And this approach still prevails very strongly in less materially developed societies and they should be our starting points for building a new world society.

UNDER DIFFERENT NAMES, but with similar objectives, quite a large number of community-based movements are active in different countries both rich and poor. It is important that they reach consensus on and a unity of purpose in regard to general principles about the means used for economic development and political organization at the level of basic communities whose choice for a no-poverty-society I have been speaking about so far. The Role of Technology in this exercise is of critical importance.

In the world today, the role of technology in economic development is rapidly changing. In the 1980s and early 1970s, technology was focussed on transferring work from human energy to fossil energy. The increased productivity that resulted led to higher wages and cheaper goods. The society of the rich prospered as long as the increased production exceeded increases in the cost of fossil fuel energy. The high price of energy, and technical innovations in the field of micro-electronics, have further changed the role of technology in society. Today technology development is directed to transferring work from human information to mechanical information stored in electronic components. This development drastically reduces labour requirements. In a recent speech, Francis Blanchard, the Director-General of the ILO, noted the following:

- A clothing manufacturer in the U.K. installed computer-controlled equipment to lay and cut cloth. This cut the work force required from 200 to two persons.
- A French firm installed robots to varnish cabinet doors. This saved

40% of the costs of varnish and reduced the number of operators from one hundred to six.

- In a Dutch warehouse, introduction of computerized stock control systems resulted in a staff reduction from 300 people to sixty-eight.

The rapid application of micro-electronic development will destroy the comparative advantage several LDCs (Less Developed Countries) hold in labour-intensive industries developed at great cost in Sri Lanka, the garment industry had a certain advantage because of cheap skilled labour. In 1981, clothing exports of third world economies accounted for 41% of the world total and was worth $17,000 million. The application of micro-electronics to the clothing industry will shift this comparative advantage in only a couple of years to the industrialized countries, leaving millions of skilled and semi-skilled workers in the third world on what is now fashionably called "extended holidays".

The so-called third world countries will never succeed in reversing this trend if they continue to depend on the Western materialistic model of development, with its technologies and political and economic structures and their clever quantitative growth indicators. We all are familiar with the number game the IMF and the World Bank play with our economies. If countries like Sri Lanka were to obtain an economic growth rate in absolute terms in dollars comparable to the rich nations, we would require an investment of capital that surpasses many times the amount of money currently available in the whole world. Those countries that followed the Western economic model now are in debt to the international financial system by over a trillion dollars!

With the publication of Dr E. F. Schumacher's *Small is Beautiful*, the assumption on which the Western economic development model was based, namely, that the best economic return can be achieved by investments in the most advanced technology regardless of the situation or context in which it is applied, was questioned. The social or ecological consequences were seriously questioned in many quarters. In particular, planners and decision-makers, governments and development organizations responded by announcing policies that would channel part of their resources directly to the poor.

Experiments began with various Integrated Rural Development projects. These were very encouraging at the conceptual level and, in effect, some integration between different sectors of rural development took place. Almost spontaneously dozens of Appropriate Technology Groups at the national and international levels sprang up and tried to find new technologies that could be applied to sustainable development. Unfortunately, lack of legally constituted and decentralized decision-making instruments directly controlled by the poor people themselves prevented the benefits from reaching them and also prevented the spiritual and cultural aspirations from becoming a part of the integrated development process. So the end result was that the already privileged people, like contractors, administrators, scholars and urban-based business community and other elite groups, continued to benefit from the new infra-structural work that was done.

The role of technology cannot be divorced from the direct control of the people who are benefiting from it, their needs and environment, and their conception of good life.

THE PROBLEMS THAT industrial societies face are caused principally by the acceptance of the ideal of a materially affluent life-style. To achieve this life-style, production had to be maintained at an increasingly efficient level using more and more advanced technology and non-renewable resources. Now it is apparent, even in industrial societies, that the benefits of such developmental approaches are accrued by only a small minority. Of course the social and environmental costs of such patterns of development, both for industrial societies as well as non-industrial societies, are well-known. The choice of proceeding with this sort of development into the future is a matter that people in the industrial societies have to decide. Already we hear of alternative life-styles, and alternative paths to development. Some of these alternatives have evolved into movements engaged in peace, ecological protection, environmental issues, and anti-nuclear endeavours.

As far as the poor communities are concerned, they do not have to look for alternative societies or models. They already are living in a society where use of non-renewable resources is minimal, damage to the environment is negligible and aspiration for an affluent living is unthinkable. If their societies are in disarray and their living standards are sub-human, the entire responsibility for that must not fall on them but on the managers of national and transnational structures who have controlled them for many decades now.

Their liberation and human fulfilment cannot be achieved by violence, both for cultural as well as other reasons. But they can be achieved by following a nonviolent revolutionary path, such as I briefly described, where the building of a no-poverty society will bring into full play the latent cultural wealth they possess.

This is the transformation of the old society to a new society in a continuum, bypassing and also avoiding the pitfalls of the modern society.

The global question before us is how the movements working for an alternative society in the industrialized world and movements like *Sarvodaya* working for a no-poverty society can join hands to build a new dynamic world culture which can confront successfully the monstrous forces of organized greed, ill will and ignorance?

Let us end with a word from Dr E. F. Schumacher:

"We can live on a small fraction of what we are living on now, as the culture of poverty, wherever it has existed, has amply demonstrated. The great thing about the really optimistic pessimists is that they are not work shy and they do not stay at the level of talk, talk, talk. They actually get their hands dirty and do some work. Let's hope we can all graduate to that class."

A. T. Ariyaratne is the founder of the Sarvodaya Shramadana movement in Sri Lanka.

Published in *Resurgence* No. 108, January/February 1984.

PART THREE

WORKING COMMUNITIES

Introduction to Rosalind Brackenbury, Elizabeth Aylmer, Tina Wood and Gerry Thompson

TALES OF FOUR CITIES

There are several reasons for placing this piece here. I think it provides a useful summary of arguments brought out in separate articles until now. The four authors remind us of the importance of a sense of place and belonging to human happiness and contentment. They emphasize the pleasure that comes from being in a place where you want to be, which gives you a recurring satisfaction.

But do you want to be where you are? For the authors of these articles, the answer is unambiguous. It is easy to feel a vicarious pleasure as they describe the joy they feel in their home towns. Rosalind Brackenbury speaks of it in terms of a love-affair with a green city. Elizabeth Aylmer describes Exeter as a friend that it has taken time to know well. Tina Wood describes a new dynamism reinvigorating an ancient town, and Gerry Thompson stresses the uniqueness of the place and people of Belfast.

It is always possible to get the impression, if you live in the UK, that all the good places to be are somewhere else — India, California, a Greek island. These pieces confirm that we have much at home that is worthwhile and worth preserving; often worthwhile because it has been preserved from the worst that some municipal planners can inflict.

There is also in all these pieces the notion of a connection with the past, of physical and temporal rootedness. This is an essentially healthy and empowering experience whose value I can attest to myself. I live in Hooton, a place mentioned in the Doomsday Book. It is near Chester, which may yet attain its potential as one of the world's greenest cities. In Chester, in the former Via Principalia, there is St Peter's Church, built on the site and with some of the fabric of the original Roman Governor's house. There is a small café and a Traidcraft shop inside, and on visits to Chester I like to visit and enjoy the satisfaction that comes from being in a building that has known almost continuous human occupation for two thousand years.

The pieces that follow also illustrate the significant point that in order to have a vibrant community it is not essential to go out and start one. There are some intentional communities for which I have a lot of respect, for example those at Findhorn and Machynlleth. But there are others which appear to be permanently gazing inward in a task of perpetual self-analysis rather than addressing the practical issues of thriving, healthy community life. I am inclined to believe that the best route to community development is through developing the natural community in which we find ourselves — that we were born into, drawn into, or work within.

TALES OF FOUR
CITIES

EDINBURGH

ROSALIND BRACKENBURY

THE CITY I LIVE IN is one I moved to from somewhere else, in a country that is not mine. I live here as an immigrant, an incomer, someone still in love with the changed light, the astonishing steepness and drama of it, the way it is so unlike anything I had ever known. My Edinburgh is still a mirror-city, in the way that Janet Frame, the New Zealand writer, speaks of mirror-cities. They are the ones in the water, in the reflection, of one's mind; related to the real cities, but different, because of the glitter of reflection on the water, because they are upside-down. They are what you have been waiting for, without realizing. In them, you glimpse your own reflection, changed.

I still cannot write about Edinburgh without evoking this quality of a recent love-affair, a new passion. True, I have now lived here for five years. But still, some mornings, am caught out by the light in the sky, the way sun splashes cobbles, the seagulls soaring over crevices in rock, and have to go out and walk about, the way I did when I first came here, unable to stay indoors, or stop exploring, or get down to anything sensible; or pretend that life here is ordinary, in any way. My Scottish friends sometimes find this odd, even funny; several of them are trying to think of ways to leave, ways to live in the country, or go abroad, or somehow break whatever link, birth or education or habit, that ties them to this hard-to-leave town.

I want to say — spend years in the flat English midlands, then, in places where you do not want to lift your head, because most of what you see is ugliness, live among red brick and under flat grey skies, where the weather never seems to change, and then see. But I suppose that what is new, different, foreign, is for each of us what challenges, what shakes us awake.

During my first weeks here, I used to dream that I was about to be sent back where I had come from; the holiday was over, the real business of life could not be here. It could not, surely, be possible to go on living in a city you can walk out of in a morning, where you can see the blue strip of the firth at the bottom of one street, with the hills of fife beyond, and the snow-spattered hills of the Pentlands at the end of another; where you can walk to see a film, or a play, or hear a concert, where you meet people you know in the streets and have time to talk, where people care about poetry and art, where you can go easily up to the highlands, or to the sea, or down to Galloway, or into the borders; where the Forth bridge, as dramatic as San Francisco's Golden Gate, leads out to all the incredible beauty of the north.

Two details about my coming to Edinburgh: years ago, a forgotten (until recently) conversation. An old friend, who had been born here, over eighty years ago. Yes, she said, Edinburgh, I can see you living in Edinburgh. At that time, I had not the slightest idea of coming here, and was simply surprised. What's Edinburgh to me, or I to Edinburgh? I had some relations here. It was remote to me as Scotland is to people living in the south of England, who believe that it takes immense effort and planning to go north and seem to think that the border is closed by impossible weather for most seasons of the year. I forgot what she had said, until I was here, and realized that my decision to stay here was the first time I had ever decided, in my life, where I was going to live. It is true for many women, that we move to places, giving up one home, having to find another, because the men we live with find work here, or there. The decision to make my home in Edinburgh, for myself, has been an important one.

SO HERE I AM, along with many other English people, living in the capital city of a country which England has colonized, suppressed, and misused. I sometimes think that the act of colonization has been like an act of desire gone wrong: that the qualities we saw in the Indians, the Irish, the Scots, were ones we wanted for ourselves, but did not know how to reach, and so tried to take by force. So brutalized and cut off from their own true feelings were the people who perpetrated colonialism, that they simply could not act otherwise; they saw what they wanted, and what threatened them, and they went for it, often with great cruelty.

Our relationship as English people with Scotland has been different, in its history, from that we have with the Irish and the Indians, for example, but there is cruelty, misunderstanding and ignorance in it, which persists and is exacerbated to this day; there is also a longing to understand, to reclaim some lost part of ourselves, to find in Celtic cultures what has been eradicated from our own. I find as a writer, living here, I come more and more back to these themes, needing to explore the relationship, and discover, here, what it means to be English, in Scotland.

It is true that, at present, England exploits Scotland; that most Scots do not want the government that has been forced upon them; that south of the border there is little understanding of Scottish life. It is impossible to write of living in Edinburgh without touching on these things; for you need to know, living here, why an English accent often grates upon people's ears, and why the International Festival is so irrelevant to so many people, and what it is that we have to learn from Scots about their culture, by listening, by paying attention, by unlearning the assumptions that we know it all. You cannot make friends from a colonialist point of view, and I have learned from living here that however liberated we may think ourselves, we English were brought up with it, it is largely unconscious, it is not our fault, but it is lethal.

I LIVE IN A large flat near to the centre of town, with a garden and with the beautiful Botanic Gardens close at hand. Many Scottish people who were born here live in crumbling tenements, still, or in ugly newish blocks in Wester Hailes, Craigmillar and Pilton. The city itself has been saved, was saved just in time in the sixties, from some of the worse things that have happened in other cities, the general gutting and rebuilding that has wrecked so many other places.

The centre of Edinburgh is, on the whole, beautiful, with old houses being restored, tenement blocks being cleaned, places which were slums, until quite recently, being transformed. But still there are many people who have had to move out of the city centre, into bad, cheap, ugly housing, for whom trips into the centre of town are expensive.

There are, in reality, several Edinburghs: the Edinburgh of the Royal Mile, Holyrood, Charlotte Square; that of Wester Hailes, out to the west, where the Wester Hailes initiative is a brilliant example of people taking charge of their own lives and getting things going, and of Pilton, Muirhouse, Craigmillar, Niddrie, where people live in substandard housing and may be taking drugs, sniffing glue, sinking into the despair of long-term unemployment.

There is the dockland of Leith, gentrified, "Leith-sur-Mer", full of wine-bars now, a northern port trying to look Mediterranean. There is Portobello, seedy as the Brighton of "Brighton Rock" with its promenade cafés and its dirty sand. There are so many Edinburghs, and all within this small radius, close together, cheek by jowl, so that you cannot forget, when you are in one world, that the others are also there.

Any guide to any city is bound to be personal, with personal favourite places as its landmarks, to some extent. I am, as I said, still exploring. But some of the places I enjoy, my own landmarks in a city of idiosyncrasies, hidden places, in which everybody has their own little beat. Views — the one from the bus at the top of Hanover Street from where you can see the hills of fife, the glimpse down the High Street of the sea, the distant shape of the Forth bridge from Cramond, sometimes like a dinosaur in the mist; the hump of Arthur's seat, multi-faceted, rearing up across the skyline from many viewpoints across the city. Shops — second-hand clothes shops, junk shops, the brush shop in Victoria Street that smells of tarred string. Valvona and Crolla's wonderful grocery full of hanging Italian cheeses to taste, grand opera and the smell of coffee, the old gramophone shop in St Stephen's Street, the second-hand book shops, countless stores of old, forgotten, curious and sometimes useless objects which fascinate me. Places to eat — lots of choice for vegetarians, with "Seeds", "The Helios Fountain" and the café at the Portobello baths, where you can sit looking at the wild sea and eat delicious home-made food. The top of Arthur's seat at any season, for the vast view and the sense of scale it gives — imagine, a city with a real mountain at its centre from which all buildings, even the most imposing, betray their flimsy and temporary nature, and the grandest city layouts look like games.

There are days and nights on which Edinburgh, to a southerner, seems grim. Days of unrelenting greyness, with the wind whipping round all corners, dire cold cutting through the thickest overcoats, nights of howling wind and blackness, when the old houses rattle and nobody wants to stir out of doors. There are also days of fresh sunlit beauty when the stone of the city looks golden, not grey, and the trees begin to show the tenderest green, and the sky is blue from horizon to horizon, and people go round looking not just pleased, but ecstatic.

I first saw Edinburgh on such a day, with rows of people stripped so sunbathe in the Prince's Street Gardens, and a sudden flare of holiday atmosphere. I was told — oh, but Edinburgh is never like this, usually; but somehow the images have stayed, and are easily conjured back to memory. It is a city of contrasts, sharp, invigorating, not always comfortable, never dull.

Edinburgh is a "green" city, in its size, its relationship to the surrounding sea and countryside, in the number and size of the green "lungs" it has to breathe with — the parks, the gardens, the Botanic gardens, the leafy walkway along the Water of Leith, the Queen's park at Holyrood, all the astonishingly varied and rich vegetation that flourishes within the city boundaries. In a city of a rational size, built on a human scale, it is possible to rediscover all the delights of city living which made Dr Johnson say of London "He that is tired of London is tired of life." True, there is noise, pollution, traffic, cramped living conditions. Country dwellers still say — how can you bear to live in town? The building site at the back of my house winds up each morning to a pitch of clanking, whirring, throbbing and hammering that sometimes makes me long for country life; but there is still the blackbird singing his heart out in a tree in the Botanics, there are the gulls floating above city streets as if this were the beach, and the vast red and yellow cranes moving in their daily ballet, set against the grey stone of tall houses and the changing, seaside sky do have an extraordinary beauty of their own.

Rosalind Brackenbury is a poet and writer who lives in Edinburgh.

EXETER

ELIZABETH AYLMER

EXETER HAS BEEN my city for many years now and although I've long appreciated the history and atmosphere, I feel, as in a true friendship, that it has taken time to get to know it well. Visitors to Exeter would find many places of interest — for example seventy-five per cent of the old city walls which surrounded the city are still visible. The serene cathedral and the beautiful buildings and gardens of the Bishop's Palace may now be seen when accompanied by a city guide as can the underground passages! A good selection of museums, my favourite being the Maritime Museum to which I dutifully took my sons only to become entranced with the "World's biggest collection of boats", to quote from their literature, and from steamers to sampans you can board the lot!

However, if a relationship with a town or city is to develop for me I must locate and test the bookshops and Dickens Centenary Bookshop at 13 City Arcade, Fore Street, owned by Roy Parry was a good start. A very well organized second-hand bookshop and once inside I lose all track of time! Roy's father is responsible for Exeter Rare Books, 12a Guildhall Shopping Centre, a splendid looking establishment with the same loving care apparent in its presentation. For a selection of new books Chapter and Verse in the Princesshay is a favourite and then there is... well, as you can see, I'm content with the bookshops!

Global Village Crafts have recently opened a shop in South Street using an entire (former) Unitarian Church for their display of crafts from third-world countries. For crafts from the west country, however, Quayside Crafts, next to the Maritime Museum, is a rickety old building in which local craftspeople rent space to display and sell their wares and, if you can make it to the top, there is a model railway. You can eat in both these places or perhaps try one of the wine bars in picturesque Gandy Street with its exclusive boutiques and gift-shops.

Having twice lately been on shopping expeditions with time and inclination to stroll along (instead of the usual tearing about gathering only the essentials) I was able to visit shops that had appealed to me.

A rewarding stop was The Soap Shop at 44 Sidwell Street. It seems that all you need to clean yourself, your clothes, the house, car, etc., is available. Although products were pre-packed, customers were encouraged to bring their own containers for refilling — thus avoiding packaging costs and the unforgivable, unnecessary waste. All products are bio-degradable, nothing has been tested on animals at any stage of manufacture and the majority of their products have no animal content.

It is an attractive shop owned by Dot Milton, a former school-teacher with a desire to run a business and a dislike of wastage and pollution. The Soap Shop was opened in 1985 and Dot Milton is already looking for prospective franchisees who would like to run such a shop of their own.

This could be a similar venture to the Body Shops which are opening around the country. Wonderful emporiums to visit where you are encouraged to pamper yourself whilst retaining care and concern for the world we live in and close links with Greenpeace and Friends of the Earth. "You will not find images of the idealized woman in our shops or on our literature" states a leaflet that I picked up and Anita Roddick, who is the founder of the Body Shop, in interview on the radio or television, is a great asset to the women's movement. When I last heard her she was denouncing the need for yet another new eye make-up product and this reminded me of a brief encounter I had, as a temporary secretary, with a celebrated cosmetic house. The whole office was in an uproar at the thought of a new lipstick missing its launch date. When I incredulously asked if it really mattered, my Agency was asked to replace me!

Then there is Greenscene, a worker co-operative organized under the Leicester Model Rules. Ray Vail, the only full-time employee of the co-operative, can be found daily in the cheerful shop at 123 Fore Street, selling a variety of "green" items but predominantly recycled paper products from toilet rolls, stationery, cards and gift-wrap through to typing and duplicating paper.

Greenscene are also wholesalers and as there is a limit to the financial support the retail side can give, they are looking urgently to expand the wholesale business.

MARTIN AND JULIA Kuhn live in Winkleigh, Devon where they cheerfully and determinedly struggle with the growing of organic vegetables, supplying shops and restaurants in Exeter and other parts of Devon. City Dropouts who farmed stock in Wales for five years but turned to vegetables as they felt this to be a better use of the land, being a cheaper and more immediate way of feeding people. I see Martin and Julia weekly, as my house is the drop point for vegetable supplies to those of us who try always to obtain organic produce. They amusingly describe themselves as "objects of merriment" with their hand-to-mouth exist-ence, supplemented by "growing" tourists in summer and Julia's part-time job painting pigs (the ceramic variety!).

Pondering on the "better use of the land" by not using it to raise meat led me to call in to Herbies, a vegetarian restaurant at 15 North Street, and have a talk to the proprietor, Tony Day. Herbies has been open for over two years and I've been going there since the "birth". It's a vibrant restaurant, serving imaginative food at very reasonable prices. I don't think Tony needs a "plug" as Herbies is a bustley place and well worth a visit. Tony buys organic vegetables "whenever possible" and is pleased to take the surplus from private gardeners. It was a joy to be assured that if he couldn't get free-range eggs, he would adjust the menu accordingly.

Paul and Vicky Campbell's wholefood shop at 8 Well Street, yielded the answer to my highest hopes. Seasons only sell organic vegetables and free-range eggs and will not even stock sugar or any products that they believe are harmful to our bodies or the environment. To talk with Vicky and Paul was rewarding; they are full of fun and vitality. The Campbells moved to Devon a couple of years ago and, having studied macrobiotics in London, they chose a house which would enable them to hold classes and weekend seminars, mainly on macrobiotics but with an emphasis on healthy living.

These are "real" people I've been writing about, not faceless organizations with dubious financial backers. People trying to make a living whilst keeping the need to care for health and the environment firmly in their minds. There will be such people in your area — find and support them. As consumers we have the power to make a difference — please use your power.

At the time of writing, Elizabeth Aylmer was a potter and member of Greenpeace.

COLCHESTER

TINA WOOD

THERE IS MUCH TALK OF the Colchester that *was* — when the Roman walls were respected, when the Franciscan Friars lived at The Old Hall at East Bergholt and voluntarily shared their garden with Spanish-Civil-War sympathisers, when the Stour Valley "Fairs" took off, entertaining thousands with a unique local blend of music, good food etc. Harvest, a wholefood shop, opened, providing food which is still of unrivalled quality and value. And two magazines, "The Grapevine" and "The Alternative Guide to East Anglia" were brought out.

But since those days of the seventies much water has flowed over the flat lands of North Essex. Now Colchester seems more like a modern version of the Roman fortress it once was. Huge bureaucratic and consumer castles are piling up around the traditional little brick-and-beam houses, and the green space on which Joe Bloggs walks his dog is more probably owned by the Ministry of Defence, which trains and houses 4,500 soldiers on its extensive properties here.

Much of today's holistic energy is coming from a new quarter — those employed in the Social Services. Young alternatives are to be found in the Health Service, the Probation Service, Social Work and Community Work.

New dynamism is also to be found in the Colchester Arts Centre, under director Anita Pacione. It is housed in a deconsecrated church, the original "wall" from which Humpty Dumpty of the nursery rhyme fell, and comprises a fully equipped stage, exhibition space, café and bar. Its scope and vision has widened, and appeals to young and old, poor and not so poor.

John Row, who runs its bookshop, told me: "We sell stuff people don't sell elsewhere. I'm creating a resource centre for black history and art; it's a struggle to get a predominantly white town to accept a *worldview* of culture."

Another powerful crux of energy is the New Awareness Trust, started four years ago by Diana Tinson, when her home was so besieged by people wanting to borrow her books on meditation and a holistic approach to life that her husband told her to "go and do it somewhere else!" The Trust presents an ongoing programme of meditation, biofeedback, electro-crystal and other natural therapies, and a lively connection with other similar centres throughout Britain.

Built as a large country house, Old Hall houses a community which has matured through exploring the seventies' idea of self-sufficiency, nine miles outside Colchester. Thirty-five adults and about twenty-three children live under one roof, the adults, in fact, mostly working outside the community to pay for their "unit", whilst some work the Hall's sixty-five acre mixed farm.

There is a down-to-earth, happy atmosphere; when I casually dropped in everyone I met was warming up for a Victorian, full-dress, Valentine's Ball, to which friends from the surrounding countryside had been invited. By organizing this and other public events, such as Maypole Dancing and The Potato Harvest, the community takes part in village life.

THIS YEAR HAS seen the first Colchester Festival of the Natural World. A barrister living near Colchester named John Jopling, alarmed at the critical state of the planet, had the idea of uniting all similarly concerned groups in a massive synchronistic action to draw public attention to all "green" issues. Young people from schools and colleges were encouraged to organize the Festival for themselves with adult guidance. A ten-day programme of events and campaigns (e.g. to plant trees and bulbs) took place in March, and a second festival is already planned for 1989. "Lack of money won't stop me doing what I want!" says John.

Resisting the ambient magnetism of all Colchester's little satellite villages, anyone in search of refreshments in town had best go to Trader's (best value in home baking) in Sir Isaac's Walk, the Arts Centre's Gingham Kitchen (vegetarian pies and huge baked potatoes), or Plimsolls in Priory Street for crunchy, fresh salads. Hungry vegetarians (and non-vegetarians) after 7 p.m. find themselves in Bistro Nine on North Hill or The Honey Pot in St. John's Street.

And if John Row hasn't put a book in your pocket, try the Red Lion Bookshop in the High Street for a wide range of wildlife books, especially for children, as well as alternative titles.

A visitor's Colchester may seem to be awake — with its new dolls-house shopping precincts, sandblasted tombstones, and the red warning flags fluttering over the army lands — but will the upsurging energies which once built its many flint and hand-made brick churches one day express a more subtle and generous illumination?

Tina Wood helped to organize the Colchester Festival.

BELFAST

GERRY THOMPSON

CONFUCIUS SAYS, "Every coin has two sides" and, "The bigger the front, the bigger the back." The better-known, "front" side of the Belfast coin is the bombs, bullets and belligerence, the peculiar entrenched stubbornness shown by parties to The Troubles, and all that negativity. This brief guide hints at something of the other side of the coin. There are things going on that are positive in themselves; but it's not so simple as "good things" and "bad things", in some strange inseparable way they all go together.

We Northern Irish people have unique qualities; we're not like the rest of the Irish, and we're not like the Scots or Welsh, and we're certainly not like the English. We're strong-minded and determined. When we decide on something, we stick to it ("Ulster still says No"). We have a rare single-mindedness of motivation — we put our opinions and our livelihood, our families and our communities, our personal safety and our actions together in one direction. And we are capable of extraordinary warm-heartedness.

These qualities can manifest in opposite ways. We can be committed or intransigent. We can be single-minded or ruthless. We can offer the warmest of compassion or the bitterest of malice, according to approval or fear. So as well as the Troubles, there is some very powerful and positive potential. There is all the greater opportunity — and all the greater need — for positive things to be going on.

THE LAST YEAR or two has seen something of a renaissance here in, what you might call, "new age" activities. It's a bit like how things were in California in the sixties, only rather more down to earth. We missed out on flower power, instead we had the Civil Rights movement, and a renewed cycle of strife. Now, all of a sudden, there's a market for positive, growth-oriented activities.

The format of such activities is different from the pattern seen in other countries over the last twenty years. The usually conservative and respectable voluntary sector plays a big part in it here. There isn't the usual setting up of "alternative" stuff and rejection of convention. The Conventional institutions are extraordinarily open, and are initiating radical initiatives. In this peculiarly hostile province, there's a unique atmosphere of co-operation between the various parties.

The godparent of the "new age" in Northern Ireland is probably the Yoga Fellowship. It's been going for years. Initially it just offered yoga in distinctly middle-class settings, but gradually it introduced not only Yoga for the People, but also a great number of other approaches to transformation, like creative visualization or healing with colour, when such things were completely unheard of. Yoga is being taken in its widest sense — it's not just about *asanas* and postures.

There are many holistic approaches to health — health of mind/body/spirit. Suddenly there seem to be lots of practitioners like reflexologists, acupuncturists, osteopaths and even Reiki people. Group activities have been sprouting up — courses and classes and workshops such as tai chi, shiatsu, Bach flower remedies, crystals and aura work. The Natural Living Centre exists as a multi-disciplinary venue for group activities as well as offering individual help and guidance, book sales and publishing.

Health food and wholefood shops are plentiful. The more central ones include Nutmeg, Sassafras and the cutely-named Beans 'n' Things. Vegetarian restaurants are thin on the ground, but there's a vegetarian café combined with music studio facility and Belfast Musicians Collective in Giro's. (On the mainland that would be called "UB40's"). It's cheap-and-cheerful. Vegetarian food without the dreaded and ubiquitous microwave can be had at Clare Connery's deli. We haven't a new age bookshop.

The physical presence of Belfast has its particular qualities as well. A lot of buildings have been destroyed, and there's a lot of rebuilding going on (goodness knows where the money's coming from. Perhaps the speculators have been to Findhorn to learn about the laws of "manifestation"!). The security forces maintain a prominent presence. On the one hand, it seems like a city at war. At the same time, life goes on "as usual". People are as cheerful as anywhere else, generally speaking. With certain reservations about not going to certain places at certain times, one feels as safe as anywhere else. Visitors are surprised at how much they enjoy their experience. There's so much they didn't hear about on the news.

The city is surrounded on all sides by green hills or heather covered mountains. It is very compact for a capital; the countryside is minutes away from the centre in a car. The Botanic Gardens makes a downtown haven of peaceful greenness, with the added attraction of visiting the warmly exotic Kew-like Tropical Palm House. The adjacent museum has an impressive display of gigantic quartz crystals. The river Lagan's scenic towpath starts close to the centre. Just above the river, on the edge of the city, is the Giant's Ring, an enormous circular prehistoric sacred meeting place, good to visit especially at the full moon and popular any night with lovers. The provincial hinterland is pretty much unspoilt countryside throughout. The whole central shopping area is pedestrian-ized (for security reasons — the terrorists achieved, in terms of progressive traffic policy, what the planners couldn't).

Belfast and Ireland are places to watch. They have influenced the world strongly in negative patterns of activity such as urban terrorist and military control techniques. But in the past, Ireland has had a wonderful, particularly spiritual influence, as in the early Christian era. Many think that this will happen again. It's an interesting case to see what the alternative approaches can come up with in the face of present circumstances. It wouldn't be the first time in history if Confucius was right and some equally powerful, more positive influence was to emerge before long.

Gerry Thompson grew up in Belfast. In 1985 he established the Natural Living Centre there, and is deeply involved in the Holistic Health movement.

Published in *Resurgence* No. 129, July/August 1988.

Introduction to Colin Hodgetts

THE SCHOOL IS A STORY

What difference does a school make to a community? And in what ways does it impact on the health of that community? Colin Hodgetts' piece reflects on both these questions.

They are, of course, questions that can be considered from more than one perspective. They can be examined in the context of the school as a community, in respect of the health of teachers and children. This approach generates questions about matters such as the role of school in a child's health, or the relative merits of small, local schools versus larger and more distant ones. Or we can consider the broader community context; how does the existence of a local school impact on the health of that wider community? How does it impact on the identity and even the survival of that community?

Two examples may serve to make the point. One is the basic matter of what children eat and when. There has been growing concern about the nutritional status of schoolchildren in the UK, with some studies suggesting that perhaps ten per cent of children no longer eat breakfast at home, and that for some the first meal of the day may be a choc ice bought from a newsagent on the way into school. It has become increasingly rarer for families to sit down to eat even one meal in the day together. One child in six may not have a cooked meal in the evening. So children, it has been argued, may increasingly engage in a less-structured 'grazing' — an often solitary nibbling at food throughout the day — rather than sitting down to nutritionally sound and balanced meals and conversation in the company of family and friends.

A recent report on children's diet in the context of school meals gave rise to a newspaper headline "Children's health is threatened by junk food diet." The report suggested that children choosing their own food at school most often buy crisps and bars of chocolate; producing, in Liz Hunt's words, "diets which are high in fat and sugar, low in fibre and some essential vitamins." When it is borne in mind that for some children the school meal is the only hot meal of the day then the health implications are considerable.

Contrast this with Colin Hodgetts' account of how children take it in turn to cook for the school, using food produced in the school garden and learning health and hygiene in the process. The children sit down and eat together with their teachers, and most children stay to lunch. Preparation and consumption are both community acts.

The second example is the emotional and spiritual quality of what happens in an educational process. All teachers are aware that they can sometimes be working with children who are emotionally wounded. And all who work with teachers know that the teachers have sometimes been wounded as well — or worn down by their daily confrontation with irresolvable professional problems. Contrast this with Hodgetts' analogy of the teacher as a sun; not selecting on whom it will shine — a timely reminder of the importance of a healthy teacher when focus seems firmly on the curriculum rather than those who 'deliver' it.

Of the many other health-related themes in this article, I think that Colin Hodgetts' account of the Small School's attitude to the material world in which the children learn is noteworthy. It is invigorating to hear of carpets, curtains and bookcases featuring in the educational thought of the teachers. And when he comments that in the Small School "we are making things to last beyond our lifetimes", he reminds us that schools are the way in which a community reaches forward from the present into the future.

FURTHER READING

Colin Hodgetts **Inventing a School: The Small School, Hartland** Published by *Resurgence* magazine.

Liz Hunt (1992) **Children's health is threatened by junk food diet**. *The Independent* Wednesday 25 November 1992.

Richard North (1987) **Schools of Tomorrow**. Green Books.

Caroline Walker Trust **Nutritional Guidelines for School Meals**. CWT, PO Box 7, London W3.

THE SCHOOL IS A STORY

COLIN HODGETTS

As Kilquhanity is one of the oldest Small Schools, the Small School of Hartland is one of the newest of the Small School movement. It has been going successfully for four years and is aspiring to gain state recognition and funding. Devon County Education Authority has assured the Small School that they will seriously consider an Assessment which has been undertaken by the School of Education of Exeter University and which is now in progress.

TEACHER: WHAT DO you want for your child?

Parent: Six O levels.

Teacher: And what if your child is not up to six O levels?

Parent: Six CSEs.

Teacher: And what if six CSEs are beyond her?

Parent: Well, I also want her to be polite, considerate, well-mannered. I want her to become a responsible adult.

Teacher: Why are you thinking of taking her away from her present school?

Parent: Because she isn't happy there.

Teacher: Is it important to be happy at school?

Parent: Oh yes. I hated school. I don't want her to go through that. She should enjoy her childhood.

Teacher: And you think she will be happy at the Small School?

THE PARENT PUTS expectations of school in conventional order in this catechism distilled from a dozen conversations, not necessarily because of a strong belief in them but because this is what society seems to expect and maybe because they feel that this is what the teacher wishes them to be concerned about. When pressed, however, it is the happiness of the child that most parents are really concerned about. Of course, the parent also wants the child to become a happy adult, which is why exams may appear important, and some schools take advantage of this, justifying present suffering by future rewards. Slog now, live later!

I am not recommending that schools become playgrounds. Ecclesiastes said, "I see there is no happiness for man but to be happy in his work" which, after consideration, he expanded to, "This, then, is my conclusion: the right happiness for man is to eat and drink and be content with all the work he has to do under the sun." I see no reason to argue with this. I believe children and teachers are at school to work. The children of Barbiana, a small Italian village, who ran their own school and taught each other, were clear about this. And they found that children who came to them from the school in the town had other expectations. "… they felt that games and holidays were a right, and school a sacrifice. They had never heard that one goes to school to learn, and that to go is a privilege." (*Letter to a Teacher*. Penguin Education Special.)

Some of our children, too, have this attitude and resent any intrusion on their playtime. We encourage work and would like this to be a happy experience for all. The requirements are a comfortable environment, relaxed relationships and meaningful activity.

IF YOU WERE seeing a school building for the first time and asked to guess its purpose, I'm sure "education of the young" would be far from your mind. Most schools are not comfortable environments. They are far from being aesthetically pleasing. What sort of society would put its children into badly maintained, uninspiringly decorated plastic boxes? Surely not one that cared about them? These buildings are far more eloquent an expression of our contempt for education and/or children than any words could be. Nor is the reason merely a shortage of money. Economy and good design can share the same bed, as the Shakers so simply and beautifully have shown. The visual appeal of their furniture and buildings derive from a spiritual commitment, not a materialist one, and therein lies the secret. 'Tis a gift to be simple, 'tis a gift to be free… and 'tis a gift our society has sadly lost.

At the Small School we believe not only that the buildings should be comfortable, but that they are themselves an important lesson in aesthetics. We use natural materials wherever possible for building, furniture and furnishings. We put carpets on the floor and curtains on the windows. At the end of each day the children tidy and hoover so as to encourage an awareness of and respect for their surroundings. The school is a pleasant place to be and has become so for a very modest expenditure. We have had a ten-foot-long bookcase made for us out of oak by John Collins, a local craftsman. It greets you, like some solid retainer, as you enter the hall. At the other end we will be building a balcony in pine using second-hand materials and MSC labour. When that is finished we will demolish what remains of the garden sheds and replace them with a workshop, again using second-hand slate, stone and wood. We are making things to last beyond our lifetimes.

In the aftermath of Chernobyl one of our pupils remarked, "So that's how it will end!" For the young the future does not stretch very far. Our stones are sermons expressing our faith in another way forward. They are a challenge to the disposable society. They also make a pleasing environment in which to work, one modelled on the home rather than the factory.

Just as in the home we look for easy relationships, so, too, in the school. If we cannot remember everyone's name without taking one of those courses advertised in the Sunday papers, then the school is too large. Small numbers does not of itself guarantee a harmonious atmosphere but makes possible the discussion of difficulties and requires people to come to terms with each other. As in a family, children learn to relate to those older and younger than themselves. We teachers have been surprised at how easily and beneficially friendships have developed between children of differing ages, as well as a sense of responsibility on the part of the older for the younger.

THE NATURE OF the relationship between teacher and pupil is determined primarily by the teacher. To be relaxed and open means, for the teacher, to be vulnerable. With teachers, as with social workers, there is a temptation to hide behind a professional mask. A primary head told me recently that she had given up living in the same village as her school as it was like being in a goldfish bowl. Only one other head present in the group at the conference we were attending lived where he worked. This is one small example of the distancing that teachers find it necessary to establish between themselves and their charges.

On the other hand, the school must not be the whole of the teacher's life. There must be room for the teacher to pursue her or his own education and interests. Martyrdom should be resisted. A good night's sleep is more important than a lesson prepared by a tired mind.

I believe that teachers must put aside their masks, for the essence of education is in the relationship between teacher and taught. It is in the silence as much as in the words, in the growth and development that happens to both.

The teacher's greatest responsibility towards his or her pupils is to be true to the self, to his or her vision. "A man must learn to be alone, he must listen in the stillness of his own heart to the wordless speech of the Spirit, and so discover the truth about himself and God. Then his work to others will be a word of power, because it is a word out of silence." (Kallistos Ware, *The Spiritual Father in Orthodox Christianity*.) Non-believers, too, may, if they are concerned with profound and ultimate matters, also learn to be alone and listen in the stillness of the heart.

Only those who understand themselves can understand others. Real teaching springs from such an understanding, for it is not primarily a passing on of information but of facing and overcoming difficulties. These difficulties may be in the subject being studied. Equally, they may be in the psychological make-up of the student. The teacher must recognize the difference between these two types of block.

It is teaching itself that reveals to us our own inadequacies and our powerlessness. It is from a base of powerlessness that we, without seeking to be, are of help. The teacher must become human, giving up aspirations to infallibility. Must, in fact, be born a child. Only the child can speak fully to the child.

THE TEACHER MUST also be like the sun. The sun does not react, does not select the one on whom it will shine. All may enjoy its warmth and energy equally. Many of the children who come to us have wounds. There is anger, perhaps even violence, at home. Perhaps their parents no longer live together. Perhaps something happened when they were small that has prevented them from developing in a natural and healthy way. It is not always necessary to know the cause. Sufficient to know the need, which is for acceptance and love in a secure and happy environment. Sometimes it is those with the greatest need who are the most difficult to approach. They are also the ones most likely to upset the group, and therefore the teacher, who must not react to become a victim of the situation but must transcend it.

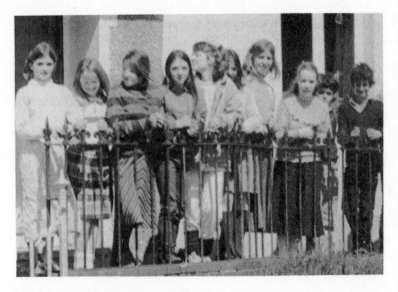

Photo by Tony Manley/ "Hartland Times"

As I talk with parents, teachers and others about the Small School, and particularly with those who are thinking of starting schools of their own, it becomes more and more clear that the heart of the school is not in the buildings, though these are important; not in techniques, though these are helpful; not in the curriculum, though this is relevant; but in the teachers themselves.

A group may sit down for years to thrash out a philosophy for the school. The group changes. Does the philosophy change? Certainly some guidelines, some general directions are important, but not too many. As Schumacher pointed out, the problems faced by such a group are divergent. The more they are pursued the more likely they are to split the group.

THE STARTING POINT for the Small School is the children and their parents. We do not really choose them. They choose us. We have said that we will take any child who lives in Hartland and refuse others only on the grounds of distance. Of course, space may soon be a problem but still geographical criteria will prevail. They will have to if we intend to be seen as the secondary school of the village.

The curriculum grows out of the needs of the children and the

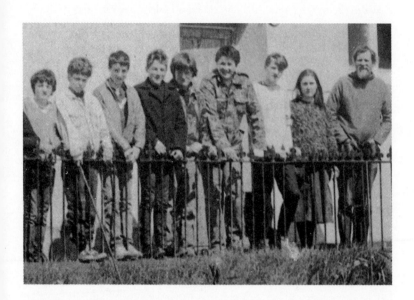

concerns of their parents. Some want exams. They shall have exams, though we try to persuade them to take only the minimum necessary. We believe that five O levels, so long as they include English, maths, a language and a science, are sufficient for entry to most places of further education.

If the Small School is to become the secondary school of Hartland, then it has to meet the requirements of all sections of the community, farmers, labourers and shop-keepers, as well as incomers with skills like pottery and cabinet-making. In responding to the demands of ecologically-minded smallholders it must not alienate conservative dairy farmers.

This does not mean that we do not tackle controversial subjects such as current farming practice, but that we try to do it in such a way as not to undermine parents and the home. I have had well-meaning colleagues who have felt it their duty, for instance, to encourage a Moslem girl to resist an arranged marriage. I believe that is wrong. It is not the teacher's task to wean a pupil from the values of the home but to respect them, explaining the child to the parents and the parents to the child.

In term time we see a child for a third of its waking week. The home has him or her for the rest. It should not be surprising if the home has more influence than the school, though sometimes parents expect us to perform the miracle that they have been unable to achieve! It is clear that a partnership between the family and the school is required, and on our part is actively sought.

Parental participation is encouraged in a number of ways. Each term we have at least three meetings of the Small School Society which all parents, teachers and pupils are encouraged to attend. All matters affecting the school are discussed. Two recent meetings have dealt with the place of sex and religious education in the curriculum. Both are potentially divisive issues. Because of our ability and willingness to look at children individually and to respect home backgrounds, parents are happy to trust these matters to our discretion. For our part we have made it clear that we cannot accept full responsibility for a child's development in these areas. The home must play its part.

MANY PARENTS ARE involved in part-time teaching, five giving a day a week. Mike teaches mechanics at his home, Pam runs textile and dairying courses at home and helps with history, English and maths at school, Philip teaches English and history and Terry teaches sewing and helps slow readers. I have a hunch that this involvement, and the fact that other children take their parents seriously, makes for a better relationship between these parent/teachers and their own children, though it doesn't always feel easy.

Outsiders also become involved. In the summer term, for instance, we have taken advantage of the Concord festival in Devon and had a two-day workshop of Ghanaian drumming and dancing with Ben Baddoo. On the second evening they have a workshop for adults to which over fifty came. We also had two workshop sessions with the Maestros steel band from Birmingham. In the evening they gave a concert in the neighbouring village of Welcombe at which our children played a piece that they had learnt earlier in the day.

The second half of the summer term was dedicated to weekly themes. In Writing Week John Moat managed to draw poems and stories of exceptionally high quality from all the children. Brian Nicholson, the head of Dartington school, was with us on the first day of Food Week and talked about growing mushrooms commercially. The rest of the week grew out of a brainstorming session and included a competition for the best plate of Danish open sandwiches, a lunch prepared by some visiting Indian students and a baked alaska, pure wickedness masquerading as a physics lesson (why doesn't the ice cream melt in the oven?). There were also individual projects on particular foods and an exploration of the moral issues connected with food and its production.

Music Week was constructed by a small planning group of students. Everyone wrote a song, many made instruments, which included an amazing ladderphone from the rungs of which were hung circular saw blades, flower pots and sections of copper tube, and some worked out a dance routine. Brian Davison, who used to be the drummer with the Nice, brought his drum-kit and a friend and held two half-day workshops. We are beginning to get rhythm!

Science Week was planned and led by Maggie Agg with assistance from her husband, Mike. It began with nine demonstrations of widely varying kinds. Groups were given the task of designing an experiment or a piece of equipment that would accomplish a particular task. We now have, constructed of wood, plastic tube, a lab stand and eight syringes, a machine that will lift an egg out of the pan and place it in an egg cup. If the egg is uncooked and fertile, then we have a solar-run incubator that can hatch it.

We rounded off the school year with a week in Guernsey camping.

When we return in September we expect to see between six and eight new faces. They won't be entirely new for two of them have been coming in on Thursdays and most of the others have spent a day at the school. Newcomers will make up a quarter or more of the school which will change it considerably. How, it is too early to say.

IT IS NOT EASY for me to answer the question, frequently asked, "How does this school differ from other schools?" Let me give one example, and as food is on my mind, let that be it.

From the beginning there has been a tradition of two of the children cooking lunch every day. This is tied in with the production of food in the garden and lessons on health and hygiene. The meals we have are wholefood, the children are charged £1 a week for them.

In the early days there was a bit of a struggle with some of the older boys. Attitudes have changed remarkably over the past two years and pupils no longer complain about their names being on the cooking rota. To tie in a subject like cooking or gardening with the life of the school brings a very important dimension of reality to the subject. The meal is being prepared for a critical clientele within strict constraints of both time and money. The absence of meat helps to keep the costs down and makes almost negligible the risks of food poisoning, apart from the moral and health issues involved.

Seeing it in action I have come to realize that skills such as bread-making, if they are properly learned, have to be practised over time. It is only after several weeks, or months even, that a young cook can know that his or her bread rolls are going to turn out well, for our bodies have lessons to learn as well as our minds.

For some people there is also a spiritual dimension to making bread. Pam, a parent who teaches smallholding skills, begins her bread-making with a minute's silence. Eating together is another activity that has a strong spiritual dimension.

Most children stay to lunch. We sit, six to a table, adults with children, and begin by saying the peace prayer. Lunch is a pleasure, not a duty, a source of happiness in our life together.

In a small village in an out-of-the-way corner of North Devon we are creating a story. We know this because we hear of it being told in various parts of the country and even across the Atlantic. Stories are powerful things. They can change the world. Perhaps ours can help to change the course of state education as a growing number of people realize they are neither daft nor alone when they ask of the system, "Does it have to be like this?" We are showing that it does not.

Colin Hodgetts is Head Teacher at The Small School.

Published in *Resurgence* No. 118, September/October 1986.

Introduction to John McKnight

UNIVERSITY AND COMMUNITY

John McKnight's interview is an appropriate conclusion to the *Working Communities* section of this book. It summarises many of the issues that have been considered in earlier pieces, and does so from a concrete and practical perspective. In this relatively brief piece he illustrates so much that is relevant to the development of healthy communities. In doing so he also models the appropriate role of the intervening academic; not full of predetermined answers to be applied before the question has been articulated, but always prepared to say "I don't know — but we will find out."

Following the theme of community empowerment, McKnight traces the steps in the process, beginning with an investigation of the real health needs of the community. Discovering that few of these needs can be addressed by the biomedical model — traffic accidents, falls, assaults, alcohol and drug abuse — the Chicago project addressed the issues sequentially. Problems of undernutrition were attacked by building greenhouses on top of flat-roofed buildings, and a surprising number of other benefits followed from this initial intervention.

Good, fresh vegetables became available at prices the community could afford; and the surplus was sold on, helping to build the neighbourhood economy. The greenhouses acted as extra insulation, so the buildings that supported them lost less heat; but the greenhouses were warm in the winter. Residents from a local old people's home came to work in the greenhouses and were reinvigorated in the process. A local youth worker who heard of their success brought up some young people to work in the greenhouses, and they became more responsible in consequence.

As McKnight comments, all these good things happened because of the greenhouse. The contrast with current top-down biomedical inter-vention could hardly be greater. But as he says, "If you want to work with communities, you have to be prepared to do humble work. You are not developing an atomic generator, important work that kills people, you are doing simple work that allows people to live."

McKnight describes another exemplary community-based initiative. This is the Learning Exchange, through which people who want to learn something are put in touch with people who want to teach it. Prospective students are encouraged to contact those who've already studied with their intended teacher, so that they can be confident they're getting somebody good.

McKnight's work is an excellent illustration of the advocacy, empowerment, and mediation approach. He and his team worked as advocates of the community, helping them find out their health needs and facilitating the development of solutions by the community. He served as a mediator between the community and powerful external organisations such as the Hospital and the University. In consequence the community was empowered by the action it took and the successes that came from this action. In my opinion there are few clearer illustrations than McKnight's of the importance of a community perspective on health, and the limitations of the biomedical model.

FURTHER READING

B. Badura & I. Kickbush (1991) **Health promotion research: towards a new social epidemiology**. WHO.

Ivan Illich (1977) **Limits to Medicine**. Penguin.

Jennifer Newton (1988) **Preventing Mental Illness**. Routledge.

Victor Papanek (1972) **Design for the Real World**. Paladin.

UNIVERSITY AND COMMUNITY

JOHN McKNIGHT

John McKnight is one of the few university professors who turn out neighbourhood activists rather than academics. At the North Western University of Chicago he is professor of urban affairs. In the biggest city of the United States he was able to start a number of projects which are examples for cities everywhere. To improve the health of the community they built rooftop greenhouses and to provide education they created a network of learners and teachers throughout the city. He visited Resurgence recently and talked about the relationship between the university and the community.

MOST UNIVERSITIES **seem to confine themselves to the academic world but you talk of moving out of it.**
When I say universities I mean large American universities like the University of Wisconsin, the North Western University where I am, the University of California, Columbia or Harvard. These universities are engaged in research and training of people to manage large-scale corporations, large school systems, large medical centres, large governments. These universities are preparing people to live at the top of the pyramid of power. When you talk to the professors they will tell you that because they are removed from the mainstream, they can be objective, they can search for the truth. But when you look carefully you can see that in fact they are not objective. They are the handmaids of the macro-institutions of our society. If you have any doubt look at their research; you will see that local communities do not exist for the universities.

But the professors will say that they work through the macro world of large governments and large corporations to benefit

local communities. The function of a university is not to serve the local communities but to influence the policy-makers.

In the United States they don't say that they are trying to direct policies to support local communities. The United States is predicated upon individualism. So, they would say more that they are supporting policies that will maximize the development of the individual, not communities. It is an important distinction. Most policy people in universities are not concerned with communities. They are concerned with only two parts of the landscape: the monumental institutions on the one hand and minuscule individuals on the other. They pay no attention to communities or neighbourhoods.

How did your Centre For Urban Affairs at the North Western University develop this idea of working in the neighbourhood?

I and some others had worked in and with communities most of our lives. When our university established an urban research centre, instead of just choosing academics, they asked two or three of us from outside too come in and become professors. I have no Ph.D., no advanced education. We decided to give it a try. I doubt very much that you can take a group of people who are pure academics and make them very useful to primary

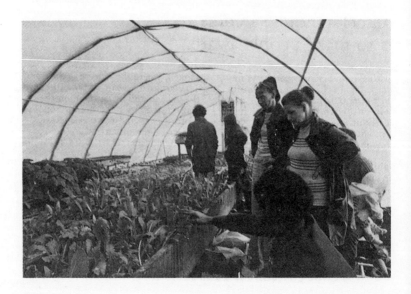

community life. Therefore they need to have somebody with them who always turns their heads away from large institutions and centres of power and turns them towards community.

Can you tell us more about your neighbourhood work?

Well, the University I am in is in Chicago, the biggest city in the United States. Here if you are concerned about communities you have to be concerned about the city. If we were in a rural area, we would have been concerned about a rural area. We are concerned especially about those people who have the least power; that means the people who are poor, minority peoples, latinos and blacks. Those of us who came from the outside came from those neighbourhoods. We have a theory that all institutions must serve communities or they are illegitimate. In fact, in modern countries like Britain and the United States this has become inverted. People say that it is the job of the communities to prepare their members to serve the institutions. If you are not ready to serve in one of these huge institutions, the community has failed in its purpose. This is the modern lie. It is a lie so large that it is now for most people the truth. We operate on the opposite premise, that the centre of the society is the community; that institutions can only be legitimate if they strengthen and serve communities rather than dominate and distort them. In that sense we see ourselves as part of a struggle to push back the institutions, and to give more room for the communities.

How do you put this theory into reality?

When I first went to university I thought that in the university there would be much that the community could use but, I found, that was not true. A community is a small group and the university is used to dealing with large institutions. We had to invent a way to make the university and professors useful. That is one of our missions, to help academics to be useful if they don't want to be slaves of the institutional spectre.

I'll give you an example. East Garfield Park was a white neighbourhood that over a period changed to a black neighbourhood. In this community, when the people were all black many institutions remained white. They served the white who had moved out but came back to be served. Two hospitals in the area were like this. So the black people formed a neighbourhood association and put pressure on the hospitals so that they would serve the black people of the neighbourhood. This was effective after two years. The hospital began hiring black people and serving black people. Later the neighbourhood association had a meeting which I attended. After there had been considerable discussion about how the hospital was now serving the community an old lady stood up and said "I don't see how this helped us." Everybody was surprised. She said "I remember how many of us were sick before. Now people are just as sick, things have not improved."

They began to discuss why that was. Was it true first of all and why? They all agreed that their health hadn't improved even though they had two nice hospitals in the community. So they turned to me from the university and asked, "Why has that happened?" I said, "I don't know. Why don't we find out?"

Now, here is something that the university can be helpful with. Because the community is not so well acquainted with how things work in this kind of institution, they thought that it must be that the hospitals are poor hospitals if they were still sick. So, we got some graduate students in sociology, economics, political science. They went into the library of the hospital and they began to take a sample of the medical records, looking at every tenth one and writing down what the record told us about the person who went into the hospital.

If you want to work with communities you have to be prepared to do humble work. You are not designing an atomic generator, important work that kills people, you are doing simple work that allows people to live. There is a very close relationship between the simplicity of the work and life. Most death dealing is complicated.

Our research showed that the largest number of people in the hospital were not there because of tuberculosis, cancer or smallpox. They were there because of traffic accidents. The second most frequent reason was because of falls; third because of assault — people being hit, shot or knifed; fourth reason: alcohol; fifth reason: drugs; sixth reason: bronchial problems; seventh reason: dog bites. We took this information back to the community. When they looked at the list they were very surprised, because that list was a list of problems, not diseases. In other words, you can't go to a doctor and get an inoculation against an automobile accident, but that is the most hazardous thing in the community. You can't get a pill from the doctor for a fall down a slum-building stairs because the landlord didn't fix it up. The doctor can't even give a prescription or an order to the landlord to fix the building. So the information made clear to them that the problem wasn't in the hospital, the problem was in the community. They understood that the health problem was their domain and they had mistakenly given it over to the medical institution. Because no matter how many times they sew up a person in an automobile accident it has no effect on automobile accidents.

We have great medical institutions in Chicago, which can never improve health because the number one killer of people between the ages of sixteen and forty-five is automobiles. So, now they had a list of the real health problems and it put responsibility back on them, not on the hospitals. They had to do something about it. When our health is placed back in our hands, all of a sudden, we will see how weak we are, because we don't have the tools, experience, skills, knowledge and political power. Where are all those? They are all in the large institutions. That is why moving towards community empowerment is a struggle about power. You cannot have powerful institutions and at the same time strong communities. You have to take power from the institutions as the communities grow in responsibility.

And you need to take some of their money.
In this neighbourhood we did a study that indicated that for every dollar in cash that the persons got just to buy food and survive, fifty cents was paid to the health service for their care. In a sense half of their income was given to medicine. If I went to the health service and said: "Tell me what would happen to the health of the people in this neighbourhood if I raised their income 50%?" They would say: "Within ten years their health would jump way up." I would say, "But you have the 50%. You have it. You are making them sick." This is iatrogenic. At the policy level the hospital is a sick-making institution. It helps impoverish the poor. It is parasitic. Now parasites can be alright. Mistletoe is a parasite on the oak tree but the mistletoe is a little plant, the oak tree is big and strong. But when you see a parasite like medical systems on poor people, that is terrible. Because the parasite is the oak tree and the community is the mistletoe.

Did you do anything to help the community to take health in their own hands?
Yes. The community asked us why people were suffering from bronchial problems, coughs, colds and flu. We said we didn't know but we would go and find out. We are in the middle of a network; that is a good thing about a university. In our network was our medical school. So we talked to people there. We were told that the most common reason for bronchial problems is because in cities poor people do not have the right food and the condition of their body is so low that they can't resist germs.

So, we had people from the medical school come and meet with the community and talk about nutrition. People said, "The main thing that we don't have is fresh fruit and vegetables. This is a slum neighbourhood, the houses are jammed together with very little ground. Then one of the people said, "Well you know most of the apartment buildings have a flat roof. Maybe we can grow things up on top. Can we do that?" They turned to me. I said, "I don't know but we will find out."

So, we went to the library and got in touch with the appropriate technology network. They said you could probably do it. You have to take earth up there but it would blow away and in the winter it wouldn't be warm, so, you would need a greenhouse. We began to explore with the neighbourhood how the greenhouses could be built and how much the materials would cost. They decided to experiment and they built a greenhouse on top of one of the apartment buildings and began to grow things. Then some interesting things began to happen. first, they got food which was fresh. That was helpful. They also grew more food than the person whose house it was on could eat. So that person could sell it in the community. This helped to build the neighbourhood economy, so it was economic development. The roofs were the major places where the buildings lost their heat; this had made the buildings very inefficient and expensive. Now with the greenhouse on top of the roof the heat which had been wasted was used to warm the greenhouse so that in winter you could grow the fruit and vegetables. Nearby there was an old people's home. They found out about the greenhouses and asked if they could come up and work in them. Many of them had been raised in rural agricultural areas. Now they could grow things and be around plants. This brought a whole new life to these old people. The man who managed the nursing home said to me, "This is unbelievable. It has changed the very nature of how these people feel about life." Then a youth worker, who was dealing with juvenile delinquents, brought some of these boys up and taught them how to work in the greenhouse and they too began to think differently. They became more responsible to each other and to the community because of their responsibilities for something natural. The food, economic development, energy conservation, bringing old people back to life and bringing young people back to the community. All of these things happened from the greenhouse. Now that is a magnificent tool. But if you go to a university, they can't help you with a greenhouse, because they will say it is too simple. If you want to build a huge geodesic dome, which will put a city under glass, they will put their minds to it.

Most neighbourhoods are not in touch with people who have telephones, who can call around the country to libraries and methods of knowing what is happening. So, we were able to find out about greenhouses and information that would start them on the way they wanted to go. We also spent some time evaluating these things — seeing how they work, why they work, so we could explain to other people if they wanted to do these things.

How were these greenhouses financed?

The neighbourhood organization has money from a trust, which it used to finance the first greenhouse. As the greenhouses developed they financed each other. You can make enough money off one greenhouse to build another. So you just need seed money to get going.

You also started a learning exchange. How did that come about?

This came from within the university. We had a couple of young people who were graduate students in education. They became convinced that none of the so-called reforms of big schools were working. Therefore they were wasting their lives getting Ph.Ds in educational administration for big schools. So they came over to our centre where they heard that we were trying to think about communities rather than institutions. One of them said to me, "Educational administration is hopeless. I'm going to drop out." So I said to him, "I have a friend who is having a seminar on education in Mexico." So he said, "That sounds interesting" and he went down to Cuernavaca where Ivan Illich was directing CIDOC. The people who were gathered there conceived this idea of learning exchange: a place where people who wanted to teach could deposit their names and people who wanted to learn could find the names of people who could teach. When he came back I lent him twenty dollars and we produced several thousand leaflets and went around the community and stuck them in mail boxes saying to people: "We are starting a learning exchange. If you know anything that you could teach, call and tell us." More and more people came forward. We built up to about 20,000 subjects that people could teach and over the years we have had thousands and thousands of people who use it. We wanted it to become economically self-sustaining, so we asked people to pay an annual membership — not much but enough for the expenses. This is a very simple device, unlike a school. It has 20,000 teachers but when you look at it, it is a small office in a church attic. It has one, sometimes two people in the office and it has three telephones. People call in and say, "I would like to learn about weaving," and you look in the card file and you see you have three teachers who can teach weaving. You can call them and see whether they want to be paid or not, where and when they can do it and whether it is a kind of weaving you want. We make a big point that we don't certify any of these teachers. Certification is the way teachers protect themselves from having to know anything. If you ask, "Which one is the best?", I say, "Why don't you go and look at their weaving, and talk to their students? Then you will really know." If I gave a certificate, you would depend on me and I would give a certificate to anyone who went to my weaving school, because I have a vested interest. Some of the graduates from my school will be great weavers, many of them will be average, some of them will be terrible, but they will all have my certificate. You may end up with a terrible weaving teacher, but you can't resist because on the wall the weaving teacher has a gold seal and a certificate from my school. I give you a great opportunity, unlike the school; I give you three people who say they can weave and you go and find out if they can. We have had only one complaint in ten years.

The learning exchange tends to be used by younger people. I think older people have been so schooled that they don't think that they could learn outside of a school. Or maybe schools made people so sick of what was called learning that they don't want to do it any more. It is used especially for learning skills, music, language, crafts, arts, etc.

Why do teachers in these areas come especially to you and why are students looking for these subjects?

I think it is because schools are least effective when you are learning how to do something with your hands. There is no substitute for an apprentice-like relationship. Therefore our learning exchange is in part an apprentice/master bank. It also operates in many other areas. There are people who are interested in teaching Greek philosophy. A person using the learning exchange could in the same amount of time as a student at high school become a hundred times better educated and for half the price.

Do you have any practical way of going about empowering the neighbourhoods, politically?

We are just beginning there. In American cities central government has all the local power and communities have none. What has happened in the last forty years is that more and more powers have gone from the cities to the state and from the state to the federal government. So we are beginning to develop a network of people who are going to lobby, to develop research, argument, advocacy for dispersing authority from the central government to the local neighbourhoods.

What areas do you want to see neighbourhood governments in charge of? Taxation?

Yes. The neighbourhood ought to be able to decide what will be done with at least a part of the taxes that come from the neighbourhood. At present all the taxes from the neighbourhood go to the central authority which then decides what will be done with it for the neighbourhood. In poor neighbourhoods there is a second issue. Taxation redistributes income so that poor neighbourhoods have extra money coming to them. But it comes in programmes: health programmes, social service programmes, child programmes, all sorts of programmes. We would like to have that money come to the poor neighbourhoods as money, not as programmes, so that the people can decide how they will develop their own community. That money could be used as investment for enterprises that would begin to build an economy that would free them from dependence on services provided by the government. In other words, the institutional servants, who are helping the poor, are really taking investment capital away from the people and using it for themselves. We say, "Don't help them. Just give us your salary and we will invest it in greenhouses or something. We will be infinitely better off than with your medical service or social service."

What about legal power?

That is more difficult. But I would like to see local communities having power to decide what shall be a violation of law in the criminal sense and what shall be the penalty. We know in our big cities that our criminal laws are an absolute failure. We are sending large numbers of young men, mostly black, away to prison where their experience is hideous and they come out angry, bitter and better trained in the ways of crime. They are then a literal menace. We have made them criminals. One way to break that is to put the authority at a local level for people to define what is allowed and what isn't. And to have community people involved in what I call adjudication. And here I can go a little further — I think the most anti-revolutionary power is the power to exile. That is, if you have a community which has a bad social order, which produces lots of people who are mentally ill, who are physically unhealthy, whose children are delinquent, or criminal and you send all of those people outside to be institutionalized, in hospitals, prisons, reformatories, then you have made it possible for the community to continue to have a bad social order. The message of this exile is: we are O.K. but those people whom we send out are bad. And the social service professional is the key person in this anti-revolutionary system. Social services encourage this exile. They say: you exile them and we will take care of them. I would like to draw a boundary around the community, and say: when your children commit crimes, you can do anything you want, except send them out. When people become mentally ill, you can't send them away; you have to look after them. You will then assume the therapeutic role which the professional now performs. Maybe you will be forced to do what you should have done in the first place. You will think, "I have so many juvenile delinquents, I can't take care of them. I must figure out why we have so many juvenile delinquents." And you know what we will find out? We, the community, make them. So, to deal with our problem, we will have to change the community. That is where true revolution starts.

John McKnight is Director of Community Studies at the Center for Urban Affairs and Policy Research, North Western University, Evanston, Illinois.

Published in *Resurgence* No. 95, November/December 1982.

PART FOUR

PLANNING
COMMUNITIES

Introduction to John Thompson

BUILDING COMMUNITY

In this section on *Planning Communities* the emphasis is on the formal planning process, with an accent on social architecture. There is a discipline called Environmental Psychology, whose focus is on the way the physical structure and formal layout of the built environment affects human behaviour. Work has ranged from the design of a hospital accident and emergency department to the layout of exhibitions. Social architecture is concerned with some of the same issues, but on the larger scale of the community.

The relevance of architecture and planning to health is evident. At the individual and family level, it largely determines the physical quality of housing stock, which a recent BMJ publication has shown once more to be very significant in physical and mental health. The physical health relevance is illustrated by the incidence of respiratory disorders such as asthma, which are associated with cold, damp conditions and poorly insulated dwellings, resulting in the growth of moulds which are associated with asthmatic attacks. The mental health relevance is illustrated by the incidence of anomie, isolation and depression associated with certain types of multi-storey accommodation.

The interview with John Thompson explores a number of issues relevant to healthy communities. He describes community architecture as concerned with an organic process as well as a product, and as being responsive to place, people and situation. The concept is illustrated with a description of the King's Cross Community project. Community representatives met with a team of professional planners to agree a community brief. This was further refined before planning permission was sought.

Such techniques for resolving the tension between developers and the community have worked before, says Thompson — in Brick Lane and Spitalfields, for example. The article ends with some suggestions as to how community-based projects can be fostered in the future, and notes that community architecture and planning are really part of thinking about Gaia; of taking seriously the notion that the environment belongs to us all.

FURTHER READING

David Engwicht (1992) **Towards An Eco-City — Calming the Traffic**. Envirobook.

William Ittleson et al (1979) **An Introduction to Environmental Psychology**. Holt, Rinehart & Winston.

Charles Knevitt & Nick Wates (1981) **Community Architecture: How People are Creating their own Environment**. Penguin.

Stella Lowry & W. F. Bynum (1991) **Housing and Health**. *British Medical Journal.*

BUILDING COMMUNITY

JOHN THOMPSON

This is the edited text of an interview by Geoffrey Cooper.

WHAT DOES THE term "community architecture" actually mean?

Well, I believe that architecture should grow out of the needs and aspirations of the people whom architects serve. The crucial question for every architect to address is therefore, "Whom do I serve?"

Do we merely serve our paymasters, are we merely satisfying ourselves and our professional peer group or are we genuinely interested in serving a much wider community — all those people who will directly and indirectly experience the environments we create? If we are interested in serving this wider community and if we respect their own particular knowledge and experience, then how can we create a meaningful role for them to play during the decision-making process?

Community architecture has as much to do with "process" as it does with "product". It brings with it no predetermined stylistic or technological intention. Community architecture is created by an organic process, unique to every situation, responding both to the nature of the people as well as to the nature of the place, the *genius loci*.

So, you are saying that architects should have a social responsibility, and that if all architects had that, then we would get much more responsive and responsible architecture?

Yes. We are an immensely powerful profession, with tremendous potential to influence not only how our environment is designed, but also, and perhaps more importantly, how it is actually created. Our analytical and technical skills form the basis of our craft — design and construction are the essential tools of our trade, but I believe we have the capacity to be creative in a much wider sense than merely producing three-dimensional forms in the sunlight — what you might call architects' architecture.

From the bitter lessons of the recent past, we have learnt that unless the environments we create are capable of being sustained by the people who actually live and work in them, they are likely to self-destruct. So, if we are to protect the enormous capital investments that are made every day in the built environment, we need to think carefully about each phase of the development process. Who decides? Who provides? Who sustains? These are all critical questions. Unless we can create physical *and* social balance, the risk of failure will be high.

Let's go on to the King's Cross project. How long has it been progressing?
British Rail started to market their surplus land, to the north of King's Cross Station, about three years ago. The London Regeneration Consortium was chosen from a shortlist of developers and the intention is that they should develop the land in partnership with British Rail.

What kind of development would you normally expect from that sort of partnership of interest?
There are really two interests involved, and by their combination they make a pretty powerful cocktail. Speculative development, by definition, exploits the nature of whatever situation it finds itself in. The more every angle is exploited, the further every frontier is pushed, the more "successful" in its terms (i.e. profit) it becomes. At the moment, the framework for speculative development in Britain has never been more fluid. The unstated rules are that developers are allowed to make their own rules! British Rail's interests are somewhat different, but they too now find themselves having to make up the rules as they go along.

With the abolition of the Greater London Council we have no central planning authority for London. The capital city of our country has no cohesive planning strategy. When it comes to transport, it is left to the developers who are trying to exploit particular sites such as Docklands, Bishopsgate or King's Cross, to try to get people from A to B, and they are expected to pay for that as well.

I understand that as far as Europe is concerned, our Government is at the bottom of the league in subsidizing railways.
Our Government does not want to subsidize *anything*! Our railways are a laughing stock (excuse the pun) compared with, say, France or Italy. It seems to me that the problem with *laissez-faire* and private enterprise is that government actually stops governing. The only point in having central government at all should be to balance the greater good of the greater number, long term and not short term, against the sectarian interest of this or that particular lobby. We have made the classic mistake in Britain of totally under-investing in our public infrastructure, of allowing the vote-catching road transport lobby to have its head and to destroy our cities, our countryside and our environment.

Without any significant public investment in transport, the developers at King's Cross must first provide profit for British Rail so that they can satisfy what they call their "operational requirements" to provide transport for the needs of London, and, through the Euro-terminal link with the Channel Tunnel, of Europe as well. The first slice of development profit, through the creation of an office city, has to go back to British Rail for something which you could argue should be paid for by the Government in any case, because it has got nothing to do with the merits or otherwise of the actual development at King's Cross. It should be seen as something which has to be weighed up London-wise or England-wise or Europe-wise.

So you have this immense pressure and conflict between the developers an d their drive for profit, in order to pay for the transport infrastructure of our capital city, and the needs and aspirations of the local community, who see the potential of the site in an entirely different way.

What are the aspirations of the local community?
Up until recently, all that local communities could do would be to snap at the heels of the developers and to chivvy local councillors into demanding more in the way of "planning gain". As in so many other walks of life, people are now actively demanding a meaningful participatory role for themselves in all the decision-making processes that affect their own lives. In the past, "consultation" was retroactive, based on conflict and not creativity. Within the community architecture and planning movement, various techniques have now been developed that allow for the active participation of local communities in a two-way educative dialogue with the professionals.

At King's Cross, the Railway Lands Community Development Group came together some time ago representing a variety of local interests. Throughout the summer, with professional technical aid, the Community Development Group has been carrying out "Planning for Real" at a variety of locations, in local schools and community centres, around the edges of the site. The process is very simple. Through using appropriate, hands-on techniques, lay communities, aided by professionals, can collectively debate, discuss and reach conclusions about very complex planning issues. The end result is a Community Brief and this tends to be very rich in its information and its detail. It is extremely relevant and provides an ideal basis from which to start thinking about the physical and social development potential of the site.

The next stage of the process is to take the Community Brief, to combine this with the local authority brief, which will have a wider perspective, to take into account any central government brief that there might be (virtually non-existent at the current time) to balance these against one another and then to produce a proposal for the site.

At King's Cross, the second stage (which will lead to the lodging of an alternative planning application in the autumn), is being taken forward by a local developer through the King's Cross Team. A Community Planning Weekend was held in September at which a wide-ranging multi-disciplinary team of professionals took the Community Brief as its starting point and, through a series of open-forum workshops, seminars and design discussions reported back with detailed proposals for all the critical aspects of the development. After further discussions and debate, these ideas will then be refined by the King's Cross Team before the scheme is submitted for planning permission.

Have these techniques been used successfully elsewhere on a similar scale of project?

Yes. On another scheme we are involved in, in the heartland of the Bangladeshi community around Brick Lane in the East End, we used all of these techniques in preparing the Masterplan for the redevelopment of the Bishopsgate Goodsyard (another British Rail site where London and Edinburgh Trust are the partnership developers) and the Truman's Brewery site (owned by Grand Metropolitan). In this case, though, community participation took place throughout the design process, and was actively encouraged and supported by the developers.

The Spitalfields Community Development Group, with technical assistance from both the private and public sectors (Business in the

Community and the Government's Task Force) drew up their own Community Plan in parallel with our own development of the urban framework for the site. We have tried to create an Urban Village of mixed uses, mixed tenure and mixed ownership, in which the community will have a long-term stake through a large slice of land being vested in a Community Development Trust, a partnership between the local authority (Tower Hamlets), the developers and the Community Development Group. Whilst no participatory process can claim to be perfect, and you can argue it either way as to whether the politically elected local authority or the Community Development Group really represents the people (or neither!), the end result has been far richer in detail and content than anything we could have produced by traditional, remote, so-called professional expertise.

What chance will the alternative scheme at King's Cross have?
Well, land values and profits are only established by the planning permissions that go with them. It is quite conceivable that the London Regeneration scheme will never get permission, or even if it does, that it may never get built. There are windows in time when political and financial forces seem to come together, and there are times when they drift apart. Nothing is static. A lot is changing right now. The alternative scheme could help to shift the agenda: it will certainly help to inform the debate. In some scenarios it could even move centre stage.

What do you think could be done to actively encourage community-based projects?
I think we have gone a long way in learning how to tap individual and collective community knowledge, and I think the time has come to examine the rules that allow development to take place. We're looking for the pendulum to swing back from being purely on the side of the developer, as it was in Docklands, back to a more meaningful level of partnership, because a partnership it ultimately has to be. If you get it out of kilter, either in one direction or the other, the results can be just as bad. If Docklands was too far to the right, then the sixties system-built estates, however well intended, were too far to the left. The missing ingredient in both cases was any form of meaningful community involvement.

If the community can join in the decision-making process, and if the community, in the widest possible sense of the word, can play a leading role in sustaining the developments that the professionals and the politicians create, then there is a good chance of creating physical and social balance. The "state" and the "market" on their own are never likely to get it right. State + Market + Community, that is what we really need. It would take a shift in the politician and legislative framework to make it happen.

Can any of this be regarded as a trend in the way planning is going?

I hope so! Community architecture and planning are really part of thinking about Gaia. We are beginning to question who owns what, why anyone should have the right to speculate on the environment because it rightfully belongs to all of us. In a way we have much more in common with the green movement than we do with the rest of our profession.

The trend I would like to see is towards responsible and sustainable environments, through the creation of development frameworks that will be attractive to both public and private investment and that will at the same time activate local commitment, local interest and, in the long term, local pride. If *that* could be achieved, then we really would be shifting the frontiers of planning into a new era.

John Thompson is a Partner of Hunt Thompson Associates, Community Architects and Urban Designers. He is Vice-Chairman of the Community Enterprise Scheme and a Trustee and Member of the Academic Board of the Prince of Wales's Institute of Architecture and Planning.

Published in *Resurgence* No. 143, November/December 1990.

Introduction to HRH The Prince of Wales

ACCENT ON ARCHITECTURE

What is architecture for? It is for human beings. Thus argues the Prince of Wales in the following piece. Citing the example of the Native American Hopi, who would consider every planning decision in the light of its potential consequences seven generations ahead, Prince Charles asserts that architecture must have firm foundations in wisdom and spiritual awareness. It may be too late to return to an Age of Faith, he suggests, but it might be possible to return to an Age of Reverence.

His Native American sources also include Chief Seattle's letter to the American Government in 1854. Its contents are well-known to many in the environmental movement, but it is pleasing to realise that in Prince Charles' original address they were repeated to a gathering of American architects. Chief Seattle referred to the web of life of which humans are a part, not the weaver, and emphasized communal ownership and therefore communal respect for the Earth.

Observing that governments and businessmen are already being forced to pay such respect insofar as they have to incorporate pollution and energy costs into their calculations, he suggests that the next logical step will be for property developers to include human and natural costs into theirs. This may ultimately lead to an equilibrium between our buildings and Nature. This could result in a wider recognition of the influence of the built environment on people's well-being, on their sense of belonging, in relationship with fellow humans — and hence on the community.

We know that the relationship between built environment and community is dynamic and direct. Healthy, happy communities are frequently those who inhabit architecture built on a human scale and which represents the community's roots in the past. Communities become less healthy when they are forced into physical constraints that destroy psychological bonds or harm physical health. The problems that follow are sometimes manifested in vandalism; an assault on an environment that is no longer seen as expressing human values or serving as a seed-bed for the growth of human potential.

The article that follows is a useful catalyst for the consideration of such issues.

FURTHER READING

Herbert Girardet (1992) **Eco-Cities**. Gaia Books.

Eduardo E. Lozano (1990) **Community Design and the Culture of Cities**. Cambridge University Press.

T.C. McLuhan (1973) **Touch the Earth**. Abacus.

Akwesasne Notes (Ed) (1991) **A Basic Call to Consciousness**. Book Publishing Co., revised ed.

ACCENT ON ARCHITECTURE

HRH THE PRINCE OF WALES

THERE HAS BEEN an exchange of architectural talent between our two countries [US and Britain] for a long time, albeit until recently on a fairly modest scale. There are one or two buildings in London which stand out by their quality and which, upon further examination, turn out to have been designed or inspired by Americans. The first store in London to rival your department stores — Selfridges on Oxford Street — has really never been bettered as a civilized piece of "retail development". Bush House — famed as the home of the BBC World Service — was designed by an American. The sculpture gallery at the Tate, which has just been restored to its full classical grandeur, is by the same John Russell Pope who is responsible for your National Gallery here in Washington.

"Exchange" has also occurred in the opposite direction — despite Thomas Jefferson's unpromising comment that "English Architecture is in the most wretched style I ever saw." I think he might have revised this opinion had he seen the Residence at the British Embassy here in Washington, designed by the incomparable Sir Edwin Lutyens. And the designer of the original Capitol — the Frenchman Benjamin Latrobe — learnt his art under England's Sir John Soane. This cultural exchange continues between us today, and is increasing — in quantity if not always in quality! There is much of positive value that our two cultures share. However, our cities also share a number of unfortunate legacies from the past, and vision is going to be needed among architects and developers if we are to be able to cope with these.

I'm sure many of you were sorry to hear recently of the death of the planner/philosopher Lewis Mumford, who drew a great deal of his inspiration from the other side of the Atlantic. I am sure that everyone here would hope that, even though he is no longer with us, Mumford's writings will continue to stimulate those who encounter them. No one, I am certain, would seriously advocate that we take this opportunity to clear the shelves of the libraries of the world of Mumford's books. Yet, unbelievably, this century began with such a plea from the world of architects and builders. One architect who made this plea was the Italian Futurist Antonio Sant'Elia, whose undeniably impressive drawings have just been on show in London. Sant'Elia was so intoxicated by the pace of change and the glamour of the machine that he looked forward to the day when buildings would last less time than we do, and each generation would have to build its own cities — the epitome of the throw-away society. If that comes about and we seem to be heading in that direction, then I shall be proud to be considered old-fashioned, reactionary, antediluvian, anachronistic — you name it!

Why *should* every generation be required to wipe the slate clean? Can't we be allowed to hold on to things of value from the past? And might we not pass on to our children something of what *we* have learned? I wouldn't agree with Mumford on everything, but he succinctly summed up my own view of Sant'Elia's mentality, and that of his followers, when he said: "If you fall in love with a machine, there is something wrong with your religion." Can I add to this that *I* feel that if you find yourself having to live or work in a building that derives its inspiration from a purely mechanical or technological source, there is something wrong with your architect? What, after all, is architecture for? Or rather, *who* is it for? The answer now — as we approach the twenty-first century — it seems to me to be the same as it has always been. It is for human beings.

I understand all the arguments about being contemporary and about the need to reflect the Spirit of the Age, but what alarms me is that the Age has no spirit. It is all matter, and therefore unable to endure. Our built environment seems to reflect the underlying misconception that we are the only generation on this Earth and that we are here to do with it as we please. We could perhaps learn from the Hopi Indians of North America whose every action was dependent on the effect it would have on the seventh unborn generation. The problem we have, it seems to me, is over the metaphor of time. Linear time justifies this modern obsession with change for its own sake, and is based on Nihilism in the sense that the line stretches to an unknown future in one direction and an unknowable past in the other. Plato and the sages predominantly talk of time as a circle — or series of circles — so that the illusion of "passing time" is the movement around the periphery of the circle. Wisdom,

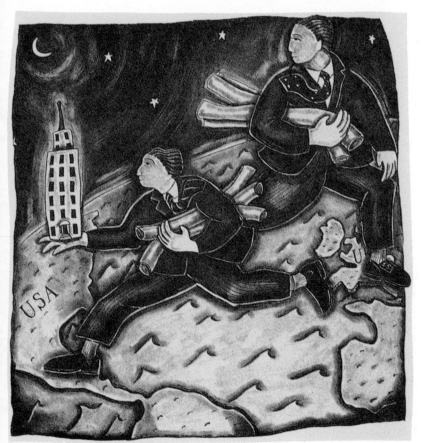

Illustration by Jackie Morris

surely, invites us towards the heart of time which is the non-moving centre of the circle. Perhaps the mounting environmental crisis the world faces will concentrate our minds and restore a degree of sanity to our outlook? Perhaps then we will begin to rediscover that human values, the things of the spirit which *are*, surely, divinely or mysteriously inspired, are the only ones which endure. They don't need to be re-invented each generation, but they *do* need to be passed on and nurtured from generation to generation.

ARCHITECTURE, AS JEFFERSON realized, is the pre-eminent embodiment of a nation's values. It never lies about where our priorities are. Ours may be an age of vast wealth, but what can we *see* of it? It sometimes seems to me that the richer we get, the *uglier* we tend to make our surroundings. What is worse, not only do we seem to have mislaid the ability to *create* beauty, but we also set out to destroy what beauty there is left in the world. The nineteenth-century English writer, John Ruskin, whose books on architecture were also highly influential on *these* shores, would have called this an age not of wealth, but of "illth" — a term he used to describe money which was poured into the production of objects, and the creation of places which diminished rather than enriched the life of man. There was, for Ruskin, "no wealth but life". Architecture began as a craft, then it became a conscious art — now it seems to be *just* a science. Surely we need to *regain* the art and the craft, and then combine them with the science.

Maybe, gradually, we are about to witness the beginnings of another age of architecture. Maybe, like an elephant, it requires a long gestation period, but as in the pachydermal case its longevity may be substantial. The time has surely now arrived when we *must* learn to work *with* rather than *against* Nature; when we can once again make places in which to live and work which are more than "machines", rather places in which we can not only *have our being*, but enrich our perceptions of what our being really is. It is in Nature that we discover the source of many of our human values.

The really interesting challenge lies in whether we can apply the "timeless" lessons of the past, and a love of natural forms, to the development of office buildings, in a city like New York or London in the twenty-first century. Why can't we create a cityscape or townscape which engenders a sense of pride and belonging, and which raises our spirits? Why on earth is it considered "immoral" in architectural circles if the outside of a building does not reflect the function of the inside? Can't we bring our rediscovered sense of Nature's value, and our human scale, to bear upon the design of wholly *new* towns and cities? It has been said to me that property developers are the "Medici of the twentieth century". Where then is our Florence? And why is a great city like London seen by our "Medici" as merely a financial staging-post between New York and Tokyo? Where has that spirit of patronage gone which always sought to offer the rarest and most magnificent examples of the architect's gratitude for a city that one could be proud of. The architecture of a country is determined ultimately by the people who *pay* for it, but it should be sure to celebrate more than just *economic* values.

There does seem precious little room in our present way of doing things for the timeless values to reappear. We might begin by paying more attention to those we build *for*. I am *not* arguing for a return to the Age of Faith which gave us our great cathedrals, but I would hope we might strive for an Age of Reverence — reverence for what gives us life, and for the fragile world in which we live.

IN THIS REGARD it is perhaps instructive to listen for a moment to the resonant wisdom of Chief Seattle who, in 1854 wrote a letter in response to the U.S. Government's proposal to purchase his tribe's territory in exchange for a regulated life on a reservation. This is what he said: "Man did not weave the web of life, he is merely a strand in it. Whatever he does to the web he does to himself... How can you buy or sell the sky, the warmth of the land? The idea is strange to us. Every part of this earth is sacred to my people. Every shining pine needle, every sandy shore. Every mist in the dark woods, every clearing and humming insect is holy in the memory and experience of my people. We are part of the Earth and it is part of us. We know that the white man does not understand our ways. One portion of the land is the same to him as the next, for he is a stranger who comes in the night and takes from it whatever he needs. The Earth is not his brother, but his enemy, and when he has conquered it he moves on."

In our own day it seems that many patrons of commercial buildings are intent on putting their "signatures" on the skyline. Much of the commercial building of today bears as much relation to architecture as advertising slogans bear to literature. The architects of "Signature Buildings" ransack History as if it were a wardrobe full of old clothes. Their buildings seldom bear any meaningful relationship to the areas in which they are placed.

I hope that when this latest fashion is played out a way of building will emerge which recognizes the *whole* picture of human life in our cities. I'm sure that our increasing environmental consciousness will lead us to that. Developers are certainly now having to take the environmental impact of what they do very seriously. One thing which growing environmental awareness is doing is that it is *forcing* governments and businessmen to think again about the way costs and profits are calculated. For example, the hitherto ignored or hidden costs of pollution and energy waste will have to be taken into account in the future. Can property developers not go one step further and begin to think more of the *human* and natural costs of development and begin to see this as economic good sense and not just idealism? We are gradually coming to realize that the long-term calculation is better *business* than the short-term.

One very important example of the challenge that I would like to see faced is the development of Paternoster Square in London, next to St. Paul's Cathedral. St. Paul's Dome is not just a bowler hat perched on top of a business-suited City. It has deep significance for both our nations — containing as it does an Anglo-American shrine to the dead of the Second World War — and is very much the heart of our own capital city. (It's also a good place to get married!) Because of this fact I believe that very great care should be taken over this site. There is a huge challenge here for the Anglo-American combination of Park Tower of New York and Greycoat of London. I am pleased to note another example of that architectural "exchange" between our two nations. However, this project is far more than just the enterprise of two developers. It should be seen as the joint effort of the people of our two nations to ensure that something of real, enduring value is created next to that great building.

We will be assisted in this, I'm sure, by the good sense and vigilance of the planners in the City of London — who are not to be won over by a few Corinthian columns. And in addition, I hope that the developer will see the need for some kind of voluntary urban framework — what has been called a *code* — which can ensure that whatever buildings are erected on the site whey will not compete for attention with each other or with St. Paul's, but will create a human-scaled, coherent and living piece of City. Think of those great towns and cities with their memorable cathedral precincts. You all know them. What makes them so special? I would suggest it is the sense of pride and belonging they engender. The civilized values they represent. The design of enclosed space inspired by what is "in the public good", as much as in the commercial interest of the business world. They raise our spirits in a way that is hard to define. Developers, architects, journalists, critics, planners want to live in such areas. People like me have parents who need to use such places for great ceremonies of state. And the buildings pay humble homage to the noble structure in their midst. So why can't we try to reorganize *our* values a little and build with this aim in mind? Why, if so many intelligent people spend their holidays in beautiful towns and cities, or in exquisite hill villages in Italy or France, do they persist in dismissing any attempt to do so as an obsession with an irrelevant past — as pastiche; as Disneyland? "What does it profit a man if he gains the world, but loses his own soul?"

Since the Age of the "Enlightenment" Man has tended to assume God-like powers over nature and his surroundings, seeking to dominate them. But we don't *have* to keep on rushing headlong into the "future" as if the whole of history were a hundred yard dash. As Mahatma Gandhi said — "There is more to life than going faster." We *can* permit ourselves to move "inward" — into tradition — "outward" — into Nature — and "upward" — to the heavens, along the way.

And it is open to us to rediscover this conception of time. Professor Christopher Alexander writes of a "*Timeless* Way" of building through which: "the order of a building or a town grows directly from the inner nature of the people... which are in it."

Our cities don't need to grow uncontrollably. We must surely accept some framework of restraint which might restore a healthy balance to our urban environment, and restore the equilibrium between buildings and Nature. These matters lead us to some of the central questions of our time. What does it mean to be *truly* human and what is a fitting way to house this human-ness? How much influence does the design of the built environment actually have on the well-being of human beings; on their sense of belonging and hence on the relationship an individual has with his fellow man — in other words, the community? And what, in the end, should be our relationship with Nature? These are *large* questions, but it has been said that civilizations are built on the questions they raise. Maybe these questions are a proper foundation upon which we can build.

It is, surely, a privilege to have the gifts of design and creativity and to be able to put them at the service of mankind. Believe me when I say that I appreciate how difficult the role of an architect is. As the progenitors of the built environment, the only public art form that affects *all* of us, you carry so many of our subconscious expectations on your shoulders. Somewhere along the line the education of architects (and developers!) has abandoned this sensitivity to the basic feelings of the ordinary citizen.

This is an edited verion of a talk given to a gathering of American architects in Washington.

Published in *Resurgence* No. 141, July/August 1990.

PART FIVE

LOCAL ACTION

Introduction to David Crouch

THE ART OF ALLOTMENTS

The section that follows is concerned with local action; with what you can *do* to make a healthy community as opposed to what you can *think*. Allotments are a good place to begin, since they contribute to human health in a number of ways, as well as serving as valuable sanctuaries for wildlife.

First, they result in a fair amount of healthy exercise, undertaken for a real purpose rather than to clock up the mileage on a keep-fit machine. Second, they provide psychologically satisfying work in convivial company; for allotment holders are friendly and collaborative people, who love to chat and to share their produce. It is hard to leave an allotment without armfuls of fruit or vegetables from two or three other workers. Third, they are a source of cheap, fresh, unadulterated and pesticide-free food, for while some allotment owners do use chemical cocktails on their produce the great tendency in my experience is towards an organic product. Fourth, they provide a convivial focus for family work. I have happy memories of picking raspberries on our allotment with the children when they were small; or of taking my elder son digging with me in the winter.

Finally, but no less important, on an allotment you can do almost whatever you please. So you see impromptu sheds made out of recycled materials. Eccentric cold-frames and complex compost-boxes, each unique, decorate the landscape and provide a vernacular and individual element in the built environment.

David Crouch's article, therefore, touches on many points relevant to our theme; and his piece is especially strong on the benefits of allotments to psychological and spiritual health. He notes the communal involvement with the land that allotments bring with them, and the opportunity they provide for exploring an alternative way of organising human relationships and values. They can be seen as a model for the development of convivial community life, and their establishment can be a significant step in building a healthy community.

It is interesting to note that in England one of the powers of a Parish Council is the provision of allotments. With the move towards parishing as an element in community development, a new parish council could well make the establishment of local allotments one of its first tasks.

FURTHER READING

John Clark (1991) **Powers and Constitution of Local Councils**. National Association of Local Councils, 108 Great Russell St., London WC1B 3LD.

David Crouch & Colin Ward (1988) **The Allotment: its Landscape and Culture**. Faber & Faber.

David Crouch (1992) **The Allotment: a Viewer's Guide**. Channel Four Publications.

R. P. Lister & Miriam McGregor (1991) **Allotments**. Silent Books.

THE ART OF ALLOTMENTS

DAVID CROUCH

WHEN CHARLES Tomlinson recalled his father working on his allotment, he called it, "A paradise; these closer communities of vegetable shade, glass houses, rows and trellises of redly-flowering beans, here grow their green reprieves for those who labour in their watch-chained waistcoats, rolled back sleeves, the ineradicable peasant in the dispossessed and half-tamed Englishman."

The allotment Charles Tomlinson was working in the fifties was above the valley of Stoke. The sanctuary of the plot influenced him. It was an escape, and carried with it deep sensory experience; the delight of growing things; the alternative experience from commercial drudgery.

The allotment attracted Colin Ward and me to research, as it contained not only all the potential for being close to the ground, but it was an experience that was widely available, and usually shared. People work the ground together on allotments; they create their own landscape around them. One in forty households do this; over half a million people. What they create is often dismissed as an anachronism, but the interest that they receive is evidence of the many more millions of families that are closet cultivators.

There is something about allotments that resembles the open field system, the communal involvement with the land; the cross-section of society and the involvement of the family discovering a whole set of human relationships that quietly competes with another set of values that dominates the everyday life.

These little plots did not emerge out of a desire to *leave* the town, but they emerged from a struggle to hold onto land, and wrest it from enclosing owners. Others claimed land from inside the city; they could not afford to leave it. From these strong political roots in the last century, it was inevitable that the allotment became significant in the way people knew each other. They share seeds, produce, and hints. For many of them, these were all they had to give. This Gift Relationship is still important in many allotment sites.

THE WAY PEOPLE have cultivated their plots over the years has produced an outstanding landscape which is unofficial and informal. The people who have long had allotments come from the "back garden" tradition of, "take us as you find us", unconcerned by the tight *presentation* of the municipal park or the studied informality that has captured the New Countryman. Edward Hyams said, "for those sophisticated flowery little plots, the work of retired ladies and urban invaders, enchanting though they often are, do not belong to the tradition of the true cottager, the cottager's garden was originally his family's larder and the vegetables and flowers mingled together in happy proximity."

Inside the plot, you experience the bulb fields of the Scilly Isles, where high hedges protect and make the secret garden. In Newcastle, and in some surviving mining villages, there is a vitality behind the corrugated iron and old doors that shut off the outside world. People work together making their land, and keeping their pigeons. Partly rusted, the slightly aged corrugated iron sheeting blends into the cooler and textured earth in an irregular and unselfconscious way. The organic growth and dynamism of the seasons provides relief and variety to the regular row cultivation that typifies the site. Along with the vegetables themselves, this provides a rich and varied texture. The allotment represents the once more leafy city. It is not urban or rural.

Away from the expectations of the house garden, and of course for those who have none, the allotment provides a wide range of the experience of working the land. For many people, the only experience of the land is as an observer; enjoying a spectacle prepared for us, distant from the conditions that produced it. In the allotment, people are actually able to feel the earth.

The allotment also provides an aesthetic adventure, whether this is in the pattern of leaves, the structural unity of the plot, the softening hawthorn hedgerow; the wind, the colour, the form of the opening leaves, and the ripening fulfilment of the fruit. There is much sensuality in the growing of things. Carol Youngson put it to me this way: "Working outdoors feels much better for your body, more vigorous than house-work, much more variety and stimulus. the air is always different and alerts the skin, unexpected scents are brought by breezes. My allotment is of central importance to my life. I feel strongly that everyone should have access to land, to establish a close relationship to the earth."

RAYMOND WILLIAMS described the different experiences in working the ground. "One cold afternoon a strip was being made ready for the first planting of broad beans. When he thought it was done, Will fetched the beans and the line, but his grandfather had started on the strip again, moving incredibly slowly, raking and raking at the earth until it seemed he was trying to change its nature. Already there was nothing larger than a marble, but endlessly, the raking and fining went on. Though he said nothing, Will doubted whether in the growing it would make much difference. It was less this, he thought, than some ritual of service. The jobs which satisfied Will were those involving an immediate, sharp effect, hauling at a grubbed root, heaving a load of leaves to the heap, forcing along a heavy bundle of sticks. To his grandfather there seemed all the time in the world, though already the blue, damp valley was thickening, and evening was drawing along the valley."

There *is* ritual in this experience, one of bonfires, a form of clothing, and a discourse; it is through the shared concerns over crops and the situation of renting land that the collective activities have become ritual. Contentious personal ideologies are challenged, and become part of allotment conversation. In turn, their boundaries are set by the seasons, the growing patterns, absorbed into the wider ritual of ground preparation and sowing.

In one allotment, seven holders had at least seven remedies for marestail between them. One turned to a flame-thrower to deal with the persistent weed, which he poetically refers to, "a web of nature's pipes". He left his plot safely that evening, only to be called the next morning by his plot neighbour. A spark must have rested somewhere on the ground, as not only had his but his two neighbours' sheds burnt to the ground. He accepted the challenge and built three sheds out of the familiar recycled materials of allotments, but a bit upmarket; floor joists from a factory, corrugated iron and shop window display units.

There used to be a familiar battle between those who poison everything on sight and those who spend a long time finding alternative methods. On some, there still is. Certainly, composting seems inevitable on an allotment, not least because of the problem of shifting bulk materials to the plot. The "saving" attitude of most allotment holders lends itself to conservation. An organic revivalist wrote in the seventies of her experience that gave amusement, but perhaps instruction, to her fellow holders. "We started the slow, laborious task of clearing the land by our eccentric organic methods, which aroused all our fellow allotment-holders to dire prognostication and much head-shaking. We dig up the sods and shake out all the surplus soil; turn them over and leave for the wind and weather to work on, then shake out more soil and pick out the matted roots. The clumps of, by then, dried grass are piled on the compost heaps and the roots left to dry out still further. They too are then composted. We can only hope that time and our better results will convince the neighbours that it should not be sent up in wasteful smoke."

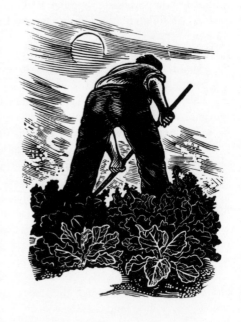

Wood engraving by Miriam MacGregor from "Allotments" (Silent Books)

In some places, people have made ecological allotments, usually organic growers, retaining trees and setting aside an area for wildlife. A place in south London has been used in this way, called Sunny Hill. And hedgehogs are endemic on allotments. Eric Simms documented twenty-three flower species on an allotment in the war years, and a reader wrote to me that she has counted nearer forty on hers. Allotment holders have joined forces with wildlife and other green groups to safeguard their sites.

IT IS THE SANCTUARY of the allotment that has attracted many artists. Miriam MacGregor has made wood engravings of people calling advice as their friends, dressed in allotment ways, batten down their shed roofs; she has also captured the expressing of a plot-holder's surprise as cattle help themselves to his runner beans. Her pictures have a beautiful whimsy. Gwynneth Leach has painted allotments full of people in Tuscany, and half a century earlier Harry Allen depicted a whole village out on its allotment. Emma Lindsay graduated from Newcastle in 1988, and had a continuing student theme of allotments in the city. There is delight in the shapes of a column of sprouts against the rich colour she saw in the profusion of sheds. In a striking series of photographs, Alec Leggatt opens up the intimacy of the "Secret Gardens" of Nottingham, and connects us with the deep relationship people feel with cultivation on these out-of-the-way plots.

Virginia Woolf wrote, in *Night and Day* of, "the idea of a cottage where one grew one's own vegetables and lived on fifteen shillings a week." For most of us, the allotment provides the most likely opportunity, whether we are living in smart town houses, crowded new village estates, or can't afford a garden of any size. There have always been people who were not natural gardeners, but for whom growing some of their own food is a moral or ideological imperative. The allotment epitomizes the Back to the Land movement of the turn of the century, and is still very much with us. It has provided a crucial dimension in the diet of many poor people.

The allotment movement has always been a part of the opposition to the alienation of urban, now almost totally consumerized, culture. Allotments have finally become the object of development; they break all the rules about profitability and privatization, although their expression of self-help is second to none. In recognition of this, the Soviet Union is encouraging a million allotments. As Richard Mabey mused, "Landowners, faced with prohibitive prices for fuel and fertilizer, realized that the most logical extension of 'Pay-and-Pick' crops was 'Pay-and-Grow'. The most eager tenants were health-food enthusiasts from North London and Stour Valley, many of whom gave up their dole to tend their vast new allotments." It may be the wider concern brought on by the food crisis that brings this about, but the return of these genuine Common Lands to many people would liberate us into more human relationships.

David Crouch is Reader at Anglia University, Cambridge and Chelmsford UK. His writing and research is about everyday culture and landscapes, including the culture and landscape of back gardens, caravans, second homes, smallholdings and intentional communities.

Published in *Resurgence* No. 135, July/August 1989.

Introduction to Frances Hutchinson

HOME ECONOMICS

Frances Hutchinson's article considers the economics of the home rather than the classroom; although it is timely to note that Home Economics does not appear in the current version of the national curriculum. This has caused concern, as it was sometimes the only opportunity people had to learn how to cook good food for themselves and their families. There are fears that dropping this traditional subject will result in even more inappropriate nutrition in young people and young families.

But the article explores wider issues than this. It focuses on the Western economic view that work in the home is ultimately unproductive, of no real economic significance; or, to put it another way, that only paid work counts. But what work is more valuable or more important than the production and care of a healthy human being?

Frances Hutchinson argues that in human life, the establishment of caring relationships has been 'the true cement between the human bricks of the community'. Health communities are composed of healthy individuals, and healthy individuals are nurtured in healthy homes. Children are particularly dependent on a sense of physical and psychological place, and Hutchinson notes the trend for childhood to have become increasingly confusing and unstable. Parents' pursuit of work may mean frequent change of home and school, and children are increasingly confined to house and television entertainment by the growth in road traffic and the degradation of the environment.

But these are still economic issues, says Hutchinson. They have to do with what we value and how we allocate resources. Currently, many matters such as the design of schools, parks, and houses are all based on the assumed centrality of the present economic system. She ends, "to be human is to be part of a human web of community and family... yet those who form this web are increasingly undermined."

This is a clear statement about the relevance of home and family to community health. Yet as Illich points out, so much of this vital work goes on in the shadows of conventional economics that it can well be called "shadow work". One feature of a healthy community is the appropriate recognition and reward of the creation and care of healthy people in the context of the home.

FURTHER READING

Mayer Hillman (1989) **'Getting About in Towns': A Diagnosis of the Problem**. *Proceedings of the Town and Country Planning Association 1989 Annual Conference*. TCPA, 17 Carlton House Terrace, London SW1Y 5AS.

Ivan Illich (1981) **Shadow Work**. Marion Boyars.

HOME
ECONOMICS

FRANCES HUTCHINSON

O NE OF THE TENETS of classical economics is that tasks undertaken in the home, and therefore lying completely outside the economic system are of secondary significance and of no intrinsic value.

Such thinking fails to appreciate that considerable areas of work have supported the economic system and added directly to material value, whilst remaining outside classical economic calculations for no better reason than pure historical accident. It further fails to account the non-economic values which motivate a large proportion of human social actions.

Economists point to the three factors of production — land, labour and capital — as the sources of all wealth. The combination of the three factors is said to result in increases in the total material welfare of human beings, bringing corresponding increases in well-being.

If we consider the factor of labour we will see that labour never did, as economists tend to assume, spring from nowhere, fit, adult, male and healthy, rattling the factory gates and raring for employment. All human labour initially emerges on the scene as a human infant, speechless and helpless, requiring several years of carefully nurtured physical and intellectual growth before it is even ready to embark upon the first leg of its years of training and preparation as a unit of labour within the formal education system. This early production and preparation of "labour", and the later tending of its needs outside school and working hours, the preparation of its food, washing of its clothes and maintenance of the domestic quarters generally, has never been included in the complex of calculations devised by economists. It has been estimated that roughly as much unpaid work takes place in the home as in formal, paid employment outside the home. The entire economic system would collapse if this work were to be withdrawn, or came to be dependent upon an appropriate economic reward within the existing system.

The present economic system rests upon the assumption that only male roles, male tasks and male achievements, dignified by the award of cash payments, and therefore capable of inclusion within the classical economic system, are worthy of note. Female tasks, traditionally undertaken in the home are, in this view, seen as merely supportive of the main male enterprise. This is to put the cart before the horse. For in human life, caring has been the true cement between the human bricks of the community. Industrial society has been built upon the destruction of these human qualities in the living community. Increasingly expensive remedial social measures are necessary to shore up the system. Highly paid experts fight a rearguard action in social, psychiatric and health care to patch up the results of inner city deprivation, drug, child and alcohol abuse.

Bee-in-the-bonnet feminists, in their haste to emulate male "achieve-ments", aided and abetted by males who have ever resented and sought to undervalue female roles, have so degraded truly feminine skills and feminine values that care of people, home and children have come to be classed as mere supportive activities. Material production of wealth within the economic system is accepted as the primary duty of every citizen, and recognition within the male status and power structures has become the sole means for expressing social concerns. Thus the woman who wishes to improve standards of education or child care must leave her own children in the care of paid strangers and seek personal and professional promotion within a career structure. This is not seen as odd. The system attributes higher significance to economic values than to human values of sharing, caring, and mutual support. Deprived of the respect and care of others, through which they could develop their own talents and abilities, those who fall by the wayside become clients or patients, the less-than-human recipients of professional care.

WHAT YOU OWN has become the sole determinant of who you are, and childhood merely a matter of passing time in preparation for participation in the adult, materially productive, world. Yet human beings are exceedingly complex beings. The care of a single human being in infancy could, on an as yet to be devised non-economic social and moral scale, be said to be at least equal to the tasks assigned to the highest-paid, highest-powered executive in the business world.

Fifty per cent of the child's intellectual potential is developed in the first five years of life, and the child's future affective and artistic life will depend upon those early foundations. Women, the traditional carers, have

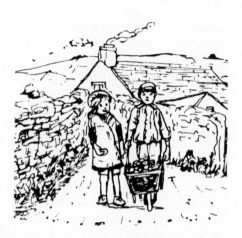

Illustration by Inger Huddleston

allowed themselves to be persuaded that "work", that is, almost any form of paid employment, is more important than the tasks of child-minding and the general care of the house. This has fundamental repercussions, which become apparent only later in life in terms of social, physical or mental breakdown.

Television is seen as a boon to overworked parents, as a way of diverting children's demands for personal attention. This is especially true where both parents undertake paid economic employment outside the home, and the bulk of household affairs have to be tackled in the "leisure" hours. Traditional child-care skills have become obsolete, as successive generations of parents rely heavily on this passive, non-interactive form of pastime.

It is being found, however, that time spent in sharing interactive toys with children, and in reading and talking to them, is valuable not only in the development of intellectual skills, but also for the growth of self-esteem and self-awareness. Frustration and alienation in adolescence and young adulthood can be linked with this early deprivation.

In separating parents and children from the home during their waking hours, the economic system is creating problems for which it has been able to deny all responsibility. Social malaise in the form of loneliness and isolation of older people is a further side effect, resulting from the economic pressures on young families to move away from the geographical locations in which the grandparents live. The full effects of the loss of natural and close inter-generational links are impossible to evaluate statistically, and so remain outside the areas of serious — androcentric — research. The concern of women at these gaps in the social network has few effective means of expression.

CHILDHOOD IN THE late twentieth century West has become confusingly fragmented. In pre-industrial times child care was not a separate adult task; it was undertaken alongside other forms of adult work. A sturdy, healthy and intelligent child was an asset to the family and to the community.

The pre-industrial child grew naturally to have a sense of physical and personal place within the household and within the community. Modern childhood is, by comparison, confusing and unstable. Parents work away from home, and from early infancy children are whisked from place to place, adjusting to different environments and different people. Home and school are in different places, and filled with entirely different people. The erosion of the countryside and the volume of traffic on the roads have led to the confinement of childhood on a scale unprecedented in the past. Present generations in their late middle age and early old age can recall childhoods where even the most inner city child could make its way to an open air and natural environment. Childhood has become a period of erratically changing but all dominating adult supervision quite different from anything which has gone before.

This may not, immediately, appear to be an economic question, but it is a fundamental reflection on the ways in which the economic system allocates resources within the community. In industrial society the buildings, institutions and structures of communal life, including the design of schools, parks and homes, are all based on the centrality of the economic system. Modifications may be sought by pressure groups, and indulged where they do not threaten the stability of the economic structures.

A feminine economics would approach the question of the distribution of resources from a fundamentally different standpoint. It has, for example, been claimed that the introduction of labour-saving devices like the washing-machine have lightened the load on the busy housewife and enabled her to emerge on the economic scene as a "worker". This train of androcentric thought fails to account the baby, child or lonely old person left out in the cold. A washing-machine in an empty house is a poor substitute for human companionship.

To be human is to be part of a human web of community and family, at the heart of which lies the essential but undervalued core of feminine and domestic concerns. Yet those who form this web are increasingly undermined in their efforts by the all-pervasive economic system. The voices of these carers have yet to be heard in Britain.

At the time of writing, Frances Hutchinson was a teacher of social science and history, living in Yorkshire.

Published in *Resurgence* No. 131, November/December 1988.

Introduction to Jo Gordon

WASTE NOT WANT NOT

The concept of the sustainable community has been introduced in a number of previous articles. A sustainable community is one which, so far as is possible, meets its own input and output needs. It produces as much of its own energy as possible, for example, and having ensured that it has as few waste products as possible takes responsibility for their appropriate disposal. As Carse observes in his thought-provoking book, waste is antiproperty, property that nobody wants to own.

Disposal of wastes — organic or otherwise — is obviously a health issue, for if done incorrectly illness will result. Jo Gordon points out that the conventional solutions have their drawbacks. Landfill, for example, has many associated problems. The amount of suitable land (if any is suitable for such a purpose) is diminishing rapidly, there may be buildup of methane gas, and leachate may contaminate the water table. I would add that the transport of material to the landfill site can also be a problem for the unfortunate people who live on the route or near the site. And incineration may be no solution; many fears have been expressed about the release of harmful substances into the air and their consequences for human health.

But is recycling the answer? Ideally, members of a sustainable community go through a cycle of four options when deciding whether to purchase some product or import some material. These are:

- refuse
- re-use
- repair
- recycle

In other words, the first step in the disposal of waste is to try to eliminate the problem by preventing it at its source; to consider whether we should *refuse* to purchase products which can only be thrown away once they have been used, or which come with unnecessary amounts of packaging. As Elkington and Hailes have pointed out, in 1986 we threw away enough drink cans in Britain to reach the moon.

Ideally, we make use of products which can be used several times for the same task or which can be put to more than one purpose. This is *re-use*. The classical example is that of the milk bottle, which on average is re-used a dozen times and then recycled. There is no reason why all drink containers could not be re-used in the same way.

Thirdly, there is *repair*. We should specify products that are designed and constructed so that when they break down, we can mend or modify them so that the scarce resources that went into their production do not get thrown away. One of the reasons I like travelling by bike is that if my bike breaks down I can almost always repair it. I understand how it works and I don't feel anxious about the possibility of breakdown (I also know that spare parts are inexpensive). This is a principle that is particularly relevant to Third World countries and their use of appropriate, as opposed to high, technology.

Finally, there is *recycle*, and recycling is the particular thrust of Jo Gordon's article. As well as considering the benefits of recycling, she considers the surprisingly low rate of uptake in the UK. Recycling schemes can be operated for glass, paper, aluminium, and textiles. Clothing can be re-used via second-hand shops.

In the present situation some products cannot be re-used, repaired or recycled — some plastics, some batteries, certain packaging. Here better product design may be the answer. But while we can't all be designers we can all be involved in recycling, says Jo Gordon, and she gives an excellent list of individual action points. It may be important to add that recycling can be regarded as an admission of failure and that it should be seen as a transitional step to a sustainable economy. Ultimately, we must not make waste; ultimately, there should be nothing to recycle.

I've been involved in aluminium and paper recycling schemes myself, and while they may start as individual action they can become a focus for community action which can lead to other sorts of healthy community initiative.

FURTHER READING

James P. Carse (1986 **Finite and Infinite Games**. Penguin Books.

Hugh and Margaret Brown (1988) **Doing our bit**. Published by authors.

John Elkington and Julia Hailes (1988) **The Green Consumer Guide**. Gollancz.

Marilyn Carr (1985) **The AT Reader — Theory and Practice in Appropriate Technology**. Intermediate Technology Publications.

WASTE NOT WANT NOT

JO GORDON

I N A YEAR the average family of four in Britain will throw away six trees worth of paper, 112 pounds of metal and ninety pounds of plastic.

As much as eighty per cent of eighteen million tonnes of waste we generate each year could be re-used or recycled, but most of this ends up in landfill sites. The availability of such sites is shrinking. Local authorities are having to transport waste over greater distances, increasing the cost of disposal. There are other problems too. Leachate from landfill pollutes water supplies and the process of decay brings about a build up of methane gas which has led to explosions.

In addition to the cost and increasing difficulty of disposal, vast amounts of paper, metals, glass, textiles and plastic are lost. These materials, if reclaimed, would have a value of £750 million.

Recycling would bring many benefits. Using resources more efficiently will reduce the production of waste, the need for landfill sites, problems of littering and pollution. Recycling also decreases the need to import raw materials, and creates a viable industry for recycling, which also generates jobs, and reduces energy costs.

Recycling can involve the whole community, encouraging an interest in a better environment, an awareness of the value of re-using materials and a feeling of making a personal contribution.

WHAT CAN BE RECYCLED? Paper, glass, aluminium and other metals, textiles and organic waste can all be reclaimed from our dustbins. Furniture and household appliances can be passed on to charities, if they are in reasonable condition.

The only national scheme for recycling at the moment is the bottle banks. There are about 3,520 bottle bank sites throughout the UK, used by nearly six million people each week, through which we recycle 14% of our bottles and jars. This does not compare very favourably with some of our European neighbours: Holland, for instance, recycled 63% of its glass in 1987.

There is no national scheme for the collection of waste paper. We consume nearly nine million tonnes of paper a year, but we recycle only 27% of this. Newspapers and magazines are collected by a few local authorities and a number of local charities, such as the scouts, church groups, and Friends of the Earth, who sell the paper to raise funds for their organizations.

Six per cent of the metal in our dustbins comes from food and drink cans. These are made from either aluminium or tin-plated steel with aluminium ends. Aluminium has a high scrap value (£350–£500 per tonne) and many local groups such as the Wildlife Trusts collect aluminium cans to raise funds. Aluminium foil, bottle tops and packaging, is collected by groups like Guide Dogs for the Blind.

Tin-plated steel cans are recovered by magnetic extraction in a few local authorities. Both types of can are collected through the Save A Can scheme which operates in sixty District Councils.

Textiles are recyclable, good quality white cotton and wool being the best materials. Rags can be made back into cloth again, used for making flock stuffing for mattresses and furniture and for industrial wiping cloths. Some local authorities do provide rag banks, or collection containers at household waste disposal sites.

Oxfam, one of our top ten retailers, have a well organized national collection scheme for unsaleable clothing from their shops. Their textile recycling centre in Huddersfield has a turnover of over £1 million a year.

Second-hand clothing in good condition does have a good market and textile merchants are concentrating more on this side of the business.

Used sump oil from do-it-yourself oil changes can be taken to some local garages and most household waste disposal sites. It is either burnt in space heaters or reprocessed to make other lubricants. It is illegal to dump waste oil or pour it down the drain and if it gets into the water supply it can cause severe damage to plants and animals, and will pollute drinking water.

THINGS THAT CAN'T be recycled. Plastics make up a third of our domestic waste by volume and the use of plastic packaging is expanding.

Plastic does not biodegrade and will remain in our landfill sites forever. In the USA recycling of plastics is well established and much more could be done to develop the potential here.

Small batteries, such as those used in radios, personal stereos, and calculators contain mercury which can be recycled. It is important this should be recovered from waste as it pollutes landfill sites and the air if incinerated. Despite these dangers there is no collection system for batteries in Britain. Holland, Germany and Japan provide collection systems for old batteries and recycle them.

An increasing amount of our milk and almost all fruit juice is packed in cartons. Fruit juice cartons are made from three layers of materials, cardboard, aluminium and plastic, which cannot easily be separated from each other and make recycling impossible. These containers cannot be incinerated as the aluminium can damage boiler tubes.

INDIVIDUAL ACTION: Use the collection facilities in your area. You can find out about them by ringing your local council.

Use returnable bottles such as milk bottles; these can be used up to sixty times.

Save clothing for jumble sales and charities.

Take waste oil to a disposal site.

If you have a garden, compost your organic waste.

Buy recycled stationery and persuade your workplace to adopt the use of recycled paper. You could also set up an office waste paper collection scheme.

Find out about local voluntary groups who collect materials in your area.

If there are no recycling facilities in your area or not enough, write to your local council to ask why more isn't being done.

We are all consumers. Manufacturers need our purchasing power. If we choose *not* to buy packaging which can't be recycled (e.g. plastics), they will begin to get the message. Don't buy packaging which you can't return, re-use or recycle. Buy well-made and durable goods which will last a long time.

Urge your local MP and MEP to take an interest in recycling.

Jo Gordon is Director of Waste Watch.

Published in *Resurgence* No. 136, September/October 1989.

PART SIX

HEALTHY
COMMUNITIES

Introduction to John Lane

COMMUNITY VIGOUR

This final section of the book, *Healthy Communities*, is a trio of contrasting examples of existing healthy communities. They contrast in two ways. One is in origin, for it is possible to distinguish between a natural and an intentional community. A natural community is one that 'just grew'; an intentional community is one founded with a specific vision and committed to a purpose. In this section we have examples of both types. The other contrast is in size; Erraid is the smallest, Davis the largest, and Findhorn is somewhere between.

The first piece is about Findhorn, and is included not only because Findhorn is a good example of a flourishing, healthy intentional community, but also because of John Lane's appropriately critical perspective. It is a perspective I shared when I visited Findhorn in 1989.

I visited Findhorn with my family, and I went there not expecting to be impressed, but I was. I remember walking along short, narrow paths to buy books at the mail order shop. The vegetation around the caravans and their extensions was hedge — or waist — high, there was trellis covered in runner beans and a glimpse of three white beehives at the end of a track. The people in the shop were welcoming and efficient. Jan, my wife, bought me a large number of books as it was our wedding anniversary that day. So I may be biased by happy recollections, but I think Findhorn is one of many possible models for the building of healthy communities. If it has limitations, they come from the nature of the particular communal vision — which is unique to them and not one that everybody wants to share.

Reading about healthy communities can be fun, and writing about them certainly is. But visiting is even better, and in the UK I recommend visits not just to Findhorn but also to the Centre for Alternative Technology at Machynlleth, in Wales. Not only is it a delight to visit, but you gain a special understanding of the meaning of sustainable community when you get out of the water-powered cliff railway and see a green line with a sign "The National Grid stops here!"

John Lane's article describes two days spent at Findhorn, and it gives an insight into the two basics of community life. One is that there has to be an utterly realistic understanding of the economic and structural basis of an intentional community. There must also be clarity about where the money comes from and goes out. There must also be clarity about who takes which decisions and how they are communicated. Findhorn, he says, is in a sense a social laboratory, and in laboratories you must always be clear about method.

In this account John Lane incorporates two useful tabulations. The first is a list of the assumptions (hypotheses) on which Findhorn is based; the second an indication of the purpose those who live there hope it will achieve. But what is important about Findhorn may be not only its methodology but the fact that it is there, it is working, and that it seems to be a healthy community. Visiting such places confirms the belief that working for a healthy community is worthwhile, and an attainable goal.

FURTHER READING

Vithal Rajan (Ed) (1993) **Rebuilding Communities: Experiences and Experiments in Europe**. Green Books.

COMMUNITY VIGOUR

JOHN LANE

John Lane visited the Findhorn Community in Scotland earlier this year [1984]. Though critical of certain elements he was moved by the spirit of the people and the clarity of their vision. Findhorn, twenty-two years old, has become a focus of community consciousness and social concerns.

The First Day

AT FIVE TO NINE we arrive by car at the caravan park. It is here, somewhere in this vicinity, that the co-founders lived and the transformative miracle began. I have never visited Lourdes but is it, perhaps, as anonymous, barren, banal as this flat utilitarian site? Ah, that such places can ever emerge from human hands, such sacred, necessary sites, not blurred by greed and vanity!

On entering the newly finished "Universal Hall" I immediately experience that visual discomfort which becomes a central concern: that Findhorn has not yet found, in the realm of aesthetics, its own particular form. Here the past has been repeatedly plundered so that amongst the echoes of Steiner's anthroposophy, Surrey's Parker Knolls and the macrame baskets and trailing plants of Haight-Ashbury, one looks in vain for something intrinsically expressive of place, of spirit and identity. The Hall lacks edge; is mushy, unwaveringly mediocre — even bourgeois; no true-born form of the soul. The newly completed Hall, eight years in the building, the focus of energy, of labour, of love, could be, I thought, a Christian Science church in Wimbledon. Had torpor set in?

But the figure on stage, an aboriginal, almost naked, is magnificent! Dark, loose-limbed, he moves with the concentrated authenticity of a natural being — a cheetah or a bird — marking out, in a trance-like dance, God's creation of the world. It is not so much a "performance" as an act of being: lithe, unselfconscious, male; a hymn of wonder and joy at the dream-like possibilities of life. And then, to jolt one sharply back into remembrance of Findhorn's alter ego, this performance is followed by another: two women, rather plump, presenting a programme of folksy "New Age" songs; sincere, no doubt, but as suffocating as a nursery eiderdown. I rush for freedom into the open air to encounter a pleasant young man: "Can I help you?" he exclaims, "Is there anything you want?" I have escaped from "love" to love.

At eleven o'clock a break in the foyer. The audience is predominantly young and feminine; but mixed; truly international. In spite of the Hall and the turtle doves I am warming up to Findhorn fast. Over coffee Sir George Trevelyan intoxicates with the life-force.

We meet Alex Walker who "focalises" the accounts office and is Chairman of the Executive Committee. Alex, in fact, is an engaging, ardent person whom any workforce would be keen to employ. He has some of the radiance of the young florentines in Botticelli's paintings: resolute, sturdy, absolutely clear: portraits of the children of the first Renaissance. Not for the first time it strikes me that a project capable of attracting and, indeed, developing this quality of person must be exceptional.

It is our first discussion and a practical one: we learn about the structure of Findhorn as a charity; of its £1 million assets; its £½ million debts; the recent (and triumphant) purchase of the Caravan Park (for £380,000); the private loans; the money still needed to complete the Hall; the turnover of some £750,000 a year. Alex explains, too, how the community has matured. "It's taken us a long time to understand," he explained, "that we have a debt, been near at times to utter shipwreck. Between 1972 and 1982 the community lost its way. Now we are aware of the need to be financially self-sufficient; that we have to pull together to solve our problems. Believe me it's much healthier."

We arranged to re-join Alex on the following afternoon and make our way to the next meeting in one of the original caravans in, as it were, the spiritual, if not the geographical, centre of the Park. Near here the giant vegetables once grew; today, there is a festive brightness of little paths, green sheds and flowers. The beauty of Findhorn steals on the mind unawares.

At noon François Duquesne and Mary Inglis welcome us into a charming room. François is French, dedicated, rather austere, in the tradition of Descartes. He has been here twelve years. Mary, also in her thirties, a woman full of courage and resolution, well-ordered, outgoing, has been here ten.

To begin with we are told some facts: that the community consists of 180 full members; that it is "governed" by an interlocking series of meetings between the Trustees, the ten members of the core group (composed of focalisers from the major functional work groups, Trustees and other members of the community) and the community itself and, too, how these groups meet, make decisions, inter-relate. We also discuss their future plans, which since the purchase of the Caravan Park, rest upon the creation of a so-called Planetary Village — a model community with its own economy based on love, the pleasure of sharing and on productive rather than wasteful activity. And as they spoke something flowered in François's pale, keen face, all will and intellect; something shone in Mary's, all gentleness and vigour. They told us:

- Our identity as persons is not vested in position; work is an act of service.
- I never doubted the park would be bought.
- Our aim is nothing less than to enable people to become whole.
- Everyone here should be his or her Trustee.
- We have had to learn the lesson that we should rely not on people, but on God.
- The resources will come when we have the wisdom to handle them.
- So long as there is a vision revitalization comes from within.
- Focusing on our problem, the debt, we never moved; focussing on creative energy we released that energy. It worked.
- There is a spirit which needs to be expressed here.
- We are working out in practice our relationship with divinity — our own, other peoples, the divinity outside us; joining together earth and heaven as a whole.
- The way our plan unfolds is dependent on each of us realizing our highest potential.

With trepidation I question them about another intuition, barely formed, almost impertinent to disclose: the lack of rigour in the community: hot-blooded and cold-blooded at the same time. Were inter-personal conflicts fully resolved? Were deep relationships actually formed? Was anger, competition, aggression, disregarded — or accepted and then, in turn, constructively transformed? Findhorn's impregnable devotion of the positive, the intuitive, the feminine, seemed to suggest an avoidance of the dynamics of confrontation. But then, perhaps, this was the inevitable consequence of being a kind of social laboratory (almost a womb) for personal and societal change? Mary and François did not disagree.

The Second Day

After breakfast I talk with the young man with whom we are sharing a bedroom; he is Dutch and "into" crystal healing. We go down into the healing room; without touching he moves his crystal over my body and identifies a particular pain. I am grateful for his gift.

Later that morning, after visiting the bookshop, the publishing hut, more people, we have lunch with Erik Franciscus, another Dutchman, a clown and a cook, the focaliser of Cluny Hill. He tells us how he holds the vision. "In the kitchen," he says, "I try to create an atmosphere like a workshop: no radios blaring, no running in my kitchen. It's you, the cook, that enhances the food, so I see that there is nothing else on my mind when I am preparing it for someone I love.

"Without a harmonious team you can't cook. So we stand in a circle, we hold hands; our whole heart and being must be present and receptive. You have, you see, to be open; to make a heart connection with the centre: to see all the negative energies being transmuted and send the Christ light to the people, the people who grew this food. I always invoke the Angel of the kitchen but not knowing from where it comes. I always can and do rely on it. The light always comes."

Suddenly, with urgency, Erik told us: "I'm not going to do anything in my life which I don't believe in. It's an insult to myself."

During lunch in the community centre I thought about what they had said. The Park has been bought; the £½ million debt is under control; the chronic insecurity, when the Foundation literally staggered from week to week, depended on nothing, so it seemed, more substantial than its faith, is now a thing of the past. The vision is a prototype Planetary Village; the realization of Schumacher's (rather than St Augustine's) City of God.

In the caravan I felt convinced; remembering the hall, I have some doubts. Might Findhorn face a crisis: to be (or not to be) what it has been: to become (or not to become) something else? The pressure to realize its vision, to broaden the base of its economy, to grow in size and influence, to "succeed" on the world's terms; these are seductive enough. But to what extent should they be resisted if their realization includes too great a degree of normalization? I wonder how it will develop in the years ahead?

We are invited to meet Nick Rose and Michael Shaw, two more Trustees. Both have been members of the community; Nick, a former Probation Officer, had come here with his family several years ago; he now lives in Cheltenham; Michael, a financial consultant, lives in London. Our conversation held against he noise of fuelling aircraft at R.A.F. Kinloss in sight of where we sat — was for me, the high point of our visit: an exquisite microcosm of Findhorn: its fabulous faith, knowing the urge of life and, no less, the pains, the responsibilities, the burden of living. They spoke of this again and again:

- Behind the world of appearances there is a greater unifying reality with which we can — and do — co-operate. The key is a spiritual focus.
- The garden as an initiating impulse was a stroke of genius.
- Findhorn is not a pattern for world development, more an alchemical retort: a point of inspiration.
- Without meditation the community would not have survived.
- Findhorn attempts to empower people to take responsibility for the planet no less than their own lives.
- Although business is at the leading edge of the cultural transformation, it is not in the "seed" of Findhorn to run businesses.
- For things to happen there must be some element of hierarchy.
- There is no tie up here between reward and effort.

On the face of it our conversation was unexceptional. But what made it marvellous and memorable was no great profundity or originality of thought but a seductive and intoxicating enthusiasm for life: the purest gnosis of "just this". No mushiness here.

Afterwards we meet Alex Walker in his neat, lucid, hut where amongst the flow-charts and the filing cabinets he tells us: "What we are attempting to do in this place is invoke spirituality; everything we do, however commonplace, is related to that. So, every morning we start off the day with an attunement, deliberately, but gently, we call upon those angelic beings who are guiding the accounts. Whatever the reality, it works. I know it works. How do I do it? Well, first I centre myself, link up with the other people in the group, and then open up to other beings of the spirit. Maybe, this way, we don't save any money, but I do it, we all do it, as a necessary part of being a human being."

Then Alex tells us about Findhorn's manifestation account, its re-investment policy and the sense of forward movement which now energizes the community at large. "You know," he says, "this *is* a wonderful place to be, though we have our problems: our debt, our personal problems, the fact we are so over-stretched. Yet, with better accommodation I can already see that I could live here for a long time. I should probably settle here for good." We say goodbye with real regret.

LYING IN BED I consider our day, its chance encounters, brief companionships, paradoxical statements; there is a lasting impression of vitality and seriousness. It would not be true to suggest that the Findhorn community "invented" the modern world — the cosmogeny of our future. Yet the people who have built, laboured, thought, lived, taught here, over two decades, have not merely challenged with extraordinary vigour the premises that underlie much of Western civilization; they have endeavoured to live, in their own flesh and blood, a new, social and psychological revolution, radical and perilous. They have striven to demonstrate what is possible when we work in harmony and co-operation with a higher order; a kinship between people and the spirit which fashions for eternity. They have happened to create a society which acknowledges the compelling primacy of love. They have sought to grow in personal insight to the higher reaches of perception, oblivious of their own pleasure and pain. And in the process they have raised something up from nothing: something subject to the severe pains and penalties as well as the abundant rewards of life; something subject to confusion, imperfection, the occasional zeal of those who preach complete tripe; yet as consistently human, liberating and life-enhancing as anything I know: a true-born fulfilment.

John Lane is a teacher, writer and painter. He established the largest arts centre in any rural area in the UK — the Beaford Centre — and a theatre company, the Orchard Theatre.

Published in *Resurgence* No. 106, September/October 1984.

Introduction to Nicola Bennett

A SNUG LITTLE ISLAND

The link between healthy communities and sustainable communities is one that we have noted already, and Nicola Bennett's article gives a feeling for what life is like in a community which has many of the characteristics of both.

The community on Erraid is interesting for several reasons. One is its demonstration of what Ivan Illich calls *eutrapelia* — a word that does not exactly mean austerity but more the avoidance of unnecessary possessions. While the marketing industry works away to persuade us that no household is complete without its own washing machine, spin dryer, television, video recorder, and so on, the community on Erraid gets by with an impressively minimalist list of possessions — one washing machine, one television, one sailing boat and two tractors.

It's interesting to read in these economically disturbed times (I'm not poor; I'm fiscally challenged!) that in 1988 the community's total income was £134,000; and that this met the needs of the ten adults and one child who composed the community; the needs of the guests, and the maintenance and improvement of buildings and land. If the creation of sustainable communities means progressively unplugging oneself from the global economic system, then Erraid may be a good model for how it's done.

Erraid is an intentional community; it is an offshoot of the Findhorn Community and shares its spiritual values while trying to practice them in a particularly concrete manner. But it has a close relationship with the natural community on the island, to the extent that friendships have been formed and the two groups cooperate over machinery, sheep-shearing, and the midsummer party.

Erraid exemplifies some of the key features of a healthy community, although clearly one that is still relatively small-scale. Each family has its own house, with room for guests (an essential item). Most of the members have acquired the fundamental skills for life on the island. The list Nicola Bennett provides is an impressive one; it includes sailing and seamanship, the care of animals, vegetable growing, fishing, cooking and candlemaking. This in itself is health-enhancing, for it would be hard to be bored with such a rich variety of tasks to undertake, and it contrasts with the alienated life so many of us live; moving papers from tray to tray or working on a production line.

Participation in work is itself health-enhancing, as Michael Argyle has shown; and reading about life on Erraid reminds me of William Morris's distinction between useful work and useless toil. Sigmund Kvalöy has written about this recently, and given a succinct description of what he calls Meaningful Work. Meaningful, satisfying work done knowing that it benefits your own community must be a vital ingredient in a healthy life.

FURTHER READING

Michael Argyle (1987) **The Psychology of Happiness**. Routledge.

Godfrey Boyle & Peter Harper (Eds) (1976) **Radical Technology**. London, Wildwood House.

Ivan Illich (1980) **Toward a History of Needs**. Bantam.

Sigmund Kvalöy (1992) **Inside Nature**. *Resurgence* 155, pp 10–12.

William Morris (1984) **News from Nowhere and selected writings and designs**. Penguin.

A SNUG LITTLE ISLAND

NICOLA   BENNETT

THERE IS AN ISLAND where there are no cars, just two elderly tractors. Where seven households share one washing-machine, one television and one sailing boat. Not only with each other, but with the 300 or so guests who visit annually. Kitchen waste goes to the animals or the garden, paper and glass are recycled , leaving only a small quantity of plastic and metal to dispose of. Nothing goes into the sea. Most food is produced on the island, the rest is bought wholesale. Visits to shops are rare and thus, thankfully, the temptation to consume is remote. In this way the community of Erraid blesses its inhabitants by making it easy for them to live lightly on the earth.

Living on Erraid means being actively aware of natural cycles. Seaweed cast up by winter storms becomes fertilizer for plants. Cabbage stalks from the kitchen are food for the cows. Manure from the byre goes on to the compost heaps. Vegetables are picked straight from the garden for each meal. The chain of life cannot be ignored, nor can the power of the elements. When force nine gales rip the lights off the cold frames, or a shower of hail interrupts planting potatoes in spring sunshine, one is forced to notice Nature.

However, to describe Erraid as a kind of ecological community is not enough. Erraid calls itself a spiritual community; an offshoot of the Findhorn Community. Erraid has emerged as a place where principles of living in harmony with nature, honouring spirit and our connectedness, could be practised in a down-to-earth way.

Erraid nudges the south-west tip of Mull, off the west coast of Scotland, and lies just across the sound from Iona. Made out of granite, the island is one mile square and feels anciently impervious to human activity. A scattering of tiny islets surround its seaward sides and a sandy channel connects it to Mull at low tides.

ON A SUNNY DAY in winter the colours are intense: the clear sea becomes a deep blue or aquamarine, the rich reddish brown of the bracken stands out against the miraculous green of the sea-flanking machair, the pinks and greys of the granite outcrops are spotted with yellow lichen and deeply riven with black cracks. When the rain and gales come the colours turn dark and you realize why the trees are small and hide in east-facing nooks. In spring and summer the valleys and crevasses are full of wild flowers, violets, hearts-ease and orchids. About midsummer pools of yellow flag irises come out and by the end of August the heather is in bloom. Seals, otters and birds live in or near the island. The wind ensures that any weather condition rarely lasts a full day, and the light changes constantly. It is so vividly beautiful that I remember feeling quite indignant on my first visit to Scotland that no one had told me about this glory so close to home.

The community lives in what was once a lighthouse keeper' settlement. They have one neighbour on the island who, with her husband and family have owned their cottage since the sixties. The settlement was built between 1867 and 1872 by R. L. Stevenson's father and uncle to serve the lighthouses of Dubh Artach. Stevenson wrote delightfully about Erraid in *Memoirs of an Islet*, and featured it less flatteringly in *Kidnapped* as the island where David Balfour was shipwrecked. The lighthouse keepers and their families lived there, complete with school and letterbox, until 1952 when the Duke of Argyll sold it to a private owner.

In 1977 Erraid was bought by two Dutch brothers who wanted their children to experience something akin to wilderness. After twenty-five years of intermittent occupation and summer lets, the gardens were neglected and the buildings in need of renovation. Hearing of the Findhorn Foundation through friends, the Dutch asked them to become custodians of the settlement: to live in the cottages for eleven months of the year and to move over for one month in the summer for the owners and their friends to have a holiday.

Over the past ten years a partnership has evolved. The Dutch arrive to find their island and settlement cared for; the houses are warm and welcoming, there are vegetables in the garden, milk and eggs in the byre, the buildings are maintained and restored. For their part, community members have the rare opportunity of living in a magical place. New developments, such as the current commitment to return an area of the island to ungrazed wilderness, are pursued by owners and inhabitants alike.

ERRAID VALUES ITS relationship with the local community. Co-

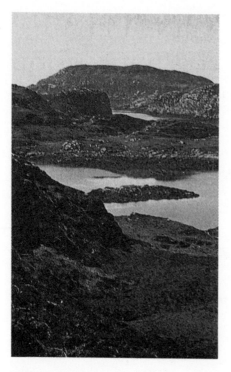

Rocks at Erraid

operation between neighbouring crofts and farms, over machinery or big events like sheep-dipping and shearing, is usual, and has been a natural way for Erraid to integrate. Personal friendships have developed, and connections been forged by children going to the local school and social events like the Christmas panto, the August show and the Erraid midsummer party. Now, and for some time, the community feels accepted, albeit, perhaps, as an unusual beast.

Membership of the Erraid community has varied over the years from six to twelve adults and one to seven children. The upper limit is naturally set by the number of houses: each member, couple or family has their own house with space for several guests.

Most of the members have learnt the practical skills needed for Erraid life since they arrived; boating and seamanship, milking, looking after the chickens, cows and sheep, vegetable growing, fishing, building and decorating, and cooking for large numbers. For the current group especially, the craft studios, where candles and stained glass are made, and the space for personal creativity are also very important aspects of the life. And all this is shared with the many people who come to see what its like to pursue a holistic life-style, many staying for a week or two, others for several months.

Each member takes responsibility for one or more areas of the work of the community. A focalizer is trusted to do their job as they see fit with the ready help of others when they want it.

Regular weekly meetings provide a space for members to share their personal and inner lives as well as their work plans. Bigger decisions are also made in these meetings and it is remarkable how easy it is to find consensus when a group is small and trusting.

The one job that all members do is to welcome guests and facilitate their experience on Erraid. Visitors are invited to join in with the community's life in the way that suits them best. Guests can relax within the rhythm of a regular daily routine with opportunities to participate if they wish.

Of the community's income 60% comes from guests, the remainder from sales of crafts and produce. In 1988 the total income was £34,500; this provided for ten adults and one child to live, for the guests who visited as well as for maintenance and improvements to the buildings and land. And no one feels they have an impoverished life; if anything, quite the opposite.

Nicola Bennett currently shares a big Jacobean house with seven other families. She is organizer of the Cheltenham Festival of Literature. She has slightly modified her article for this collection.

Published in *Resurgence* No. 140, May/June 1990.

Introduction to Richard St George

NO MEAN CITY

Richard St George's piece concludes the section and this book. Findhorn is a large, well-established intentional community and Erraid a small, younger intentional community in the process of integration with a natural community. In contrast Davis is an illuminating example of a large natural community that displays most of the features of healthy community. Which it not to say that it hasn't been without some intentional planning to make it that way.

Davis is located in California, near Sacramento. It is unusual in that it has no slums, no ghettos, low unemployment, the lowest crime rate in the USA, but a high level of environmental awareness.

How did it get that way? In the 1960s, during a period of rapid city growth, students at the locally-based University of California Faculty of Agriculture joined together to form the Greater Davis Research and Planning Group. They came up with an alternative plan for Davis which has been working ever since.

Some of the plan's ideas are classically simple. During the energy crisis of the early 1970s they planted 17,000 trees in front of houses and car parks to reduce the need for air conditioning in cars and homes. No buildings are allowed to grow higher than trees; houses can go up to two storeys, offices to four. Better standards of thermal insulation in new buildings have cut energy consumption.

The people of Davis look after their land. Chemical fertilisers are discouraged, gardens are used more for vegetables than flowers, and allotments are available. The farmers' market has encouraged the local supply of local demand, and as the consumption of fresh food has gone up, that of frozen food has gone down. Recycling is encouraged; and pre-sorted recyclable material is collected from outside people's homes. Even clothes are recycled.

Bicycles are popular in Davis; there are 40,000 bikes and 9,000 cars. This may be because cyclists have right of way everywhere and 70 km of bike lanes or cycleways to ride on.

It's interesting to speculate about why Davis has developed the way it has. Part of it may result from the citizen's commitment to participative local democracy; part perhaps from the large student population. In 1992 I visited Tubingen in South Germany, which has like Davis a large number of students and a tradition of local action.

Tubingen is also characterised by traffic calming, cycle use, and a harmonious lifestyle.

The example of Davis and other places like it is important, because it meets the objection that healthy communities are utopian fictions. There is a place for utopian fiction on this theme, and LeGuin and Piercy have both produced good books to prove it. But Davis is a real city in a real world, a Healthy City as the WHO might put it, and its existence shows us that the attainment of healthy communities is possible as well as essential. And a recurrent theme of this book is that healthy communities contribute not just to the health of humans, but are intimately linked to the health of the planet.

In a letter Richard St. George says "I should like to point out that since *No Mean City* was published, a couple of people have told me that it is Davis as seen through rose-tinted glasses!" But he adds that in one development in Davis — Village Homes — houses now change hands for five times the selling price when they were built ten years before. As prices in other non-ecological developments nearby have actually gone down, "they must be doing something right."

FURTHER READING

John Ashton (Ed) (1992) **Healthy Cities**. Open University Press.

Ursula LeGuin (1988) **Always coming home**. Grafton Books.

Marge Piercey (1978) **Woman on the Edge of Time**. The Women's Press.

World Health Organization (1985) **Targets for Health for All**. WHO.

NO MEAN CITY

RICHARD ST. GEORGE

I T IS OFTEN SAID that we live in an escapist society. Perhaps one
example of this is that we holiday in the country to run away from
our urban hells. But there is a town in California where substantially
fewer of its inhabitants holiday away. There is no need to. They like
being where they live. Why? What is so special about this town called
Davis, near Sacramento? Last year Willem Hoogendijk, Professor of
Environmental Education in Holland, gave me a videoed copy of a
documentary shown on West German television titled Eco-City Davis. It
is inspiring viewing.

Davis is home to the University of California's Faculty of Agriculture
and during the fifties and sixties the town's population expanded rapidly.
Students and worried townspeople got together to found the Greater
Davis Research and Planning Group. The aim was to preserve the town's
identity and check further urban sprawl. Working with the Low Energy
Research Group they came up with an alternative local plan. Riding on
this "Green Ticket" three students were elected to seats on the local
council. One of those original students, Bill Carter, is now the mayor.

Much has happened since to put Davis on the map and planning
experts and students travel worldwide to visit the "alternative city". Davis
has received two awards for its environmentally conscious thinking. It is
the only city in the USA without slums, without ghettos, has the lowest
number of unemployed and has only half of the TV consumption of the
American population in general. Not surprisingly Davis has the lowest
crime rate in the States. In fact the Davis community has dismantled just
about every preconception there is concerning American life-styles.

The early legislation, some enacted prior to the 1974 energy crisis,
concerned the use of energy. Seventeen thousand trees were planted, one
in front of every house and parking lot, to give shade and natural cool.
This did away with the need for energy consuming air-conditioning in
the suburbs and shopping centres. Planting all car-parks with shade trees

broke another Californian habit — that of keeping parked cars running to keep the air-conditioning going. The air pollution dropped, as did the number of victims of air-conditioning-related illnesses.

Next to receive attention were the local building by-laws. No buildings were allowed higher than the trees. Houses are restricted to two storeys and business premises to four. New building regulations demanded better standards of insulation, double-glazing, detailed sealing and solar heating of water. Domestic energy consumption dropped to a third of that in the old houses. Initially there was resistance from the developers who complained about the extra costs involved and keeping within their budgets. However, the new homes worked, were cheaper to run and sold well. The builders were convinced and have since become the greatest evangelists for the new methods. They are pressing the State to introduce the Davis regulations throughout California.

Davis survived the 1974 fuel crisis in much better shape than nearby communities and this reinforced the political will to create and apply new legislation. The population became convinced that it was possible to save energy without having to give anything up and within a few years energy consumption in Davis had dropped by a half. New developments now concentrate on passive solar design and it is hoped that by the end of the century Davis will draw half of its energy from the sun. Davis must be unique as the only town where one's energy consumption is a major topic of conversation at coffee mornings and drinks parties. Even hanging out one's washing is back in fashion. It is more hygienic and cheaper than dryers and saves energy. That's one cultural taboo out the window.

Land use is a major concern and a denser building ratio has been imposed on new developments to save the fertile land. Two to three harvests a year can be obtained without the use of chemical fertilizers which are discouraged. Gardens are used more for growing vegetables than lawns. Allotments are available for flat owners with no garden of their own. A 40 square metres plot can be rented for $12 a year which if properly used will provide a couple with 70% of their fruit and vegetables. Composting is encouraged so that the water-retention capacity of the soil is enhanced. Surprisingly water consumption in Davis is low despite the Californian sun. There is a twice weekly farmers market and this has encouraged the local farms to supply the local demand. The ecological motto is "Local Supply stimulates Local Growth." As the consumption of fresh locally produced food has gone up so the consumption of frozen, tinned and processed food trucked in from outside the region has gone down. Previously most food consumed in

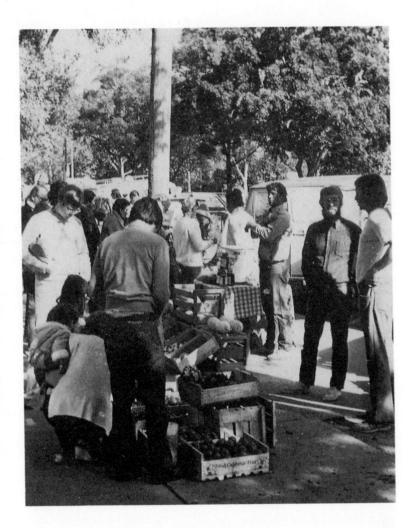

Davis was frozen so yet another ingrained habit gets knocked on the head.

Recycling is another priority. To begin with citizens had to take their bottles, tins, paper and cardboard to collection points but this met with only a half-hearted response. Now all the material is collected from the streets by specially designed dustcarts and 70% of the population now voluntarily sort their rubbish for recycling. The recycling scheme provides jobs and makes a profit for the City Treasury. The American taboo about wearing second-hand clothes has also gone by the board in Davis where there is a second-hand clothes market. The clothes are collected by volunteers and dry-cleaned before being offered for sale. The profits again go into the City Treasury's coffers. Bang goes the Throw Away Society.

THE MOST VISIBLE change in Davis (apart from its leafy streets) has earned it its reputation as the eco-city of the USA. That is its love affair with the bicycle. There is a population of 40,000 bicycles for only 9,000 cars. Cyclists have the right of way everywhere and there is even a unit of cycle police to regulate the bicycle traffic. During the mid-seventies the student eco-freaks started to spurn the motor car in favour of bicycles. However, there were many accidents and so local legislation was enacted to remove bicycles from the traffic where possible. There are now 42 kilometres of bike lanes in the city and a further 28 kilometres of cycleways in the suburbs. Busy interchanges have been modified to separate off the cyclists. Cycle traffic lights and signs warn where cars and cycles meet. Since 150 bicycles can be parked in the space allotted to twenty cars, now even the student car-park has been grassed over. So it is possible to divorce Americans from their motors!!

However, the most radical innovation in Davis is also the least immediately apparent. It comes not from its energy, transport or recycling systems. As is often the case it is a social change that has the most profound effect. In this case the organization of local government, "Less administration, more democracy" is the motto and no decision is made without a public hearing. Every inhabitant is invited to influence decisions. A step in a truly democratic process to be involved and informed which strengthens the community spirit and the feeling of responsibility of one for all. Even the arrangement of the council chamber reflects this. Most north American councils sit at a round table away from the public galleries to which the public are allowed as silent observers. In contrast at Davis, the council members sit in a semi-circle facing the public galleries from which comments and suggestions can be considered.

Not surprisingly the citizens don't want to see this local democracy eroded. The town now has a population of 40,000 and they hope to be able to restrict further growth to a limit of 50,000. Beyond that they believe their system of open local government would break down. They are encouraging the State of California to divert further development to new Davis-sized towns in the foothills and not on the surrounding agricultural land which they consider much too precious to be used as building plots.

Attitudes to change have been radically altered. In the early days when the student councillors argued for alternative planning from the recently introduced galleries, there were angry exchanges. There was a great deal of resistance to the new ideas, but as the advantages of the legislation have become apparent, further changes have been supported and opposition has lessened. These days the emphasis is on improving the ecological successes rather than controversy. Everyone now accepts that environmental change can take place without loss of convenience, comfort or any other measure of standard of living.

Nor has Davis become smug about its achievements. Perhaps because of the type of people attracted to Davis, it has none of the parochialism so common in small-town America. There is an exchange programme with Russian students supported by the city. The level of public interest in issues such as nuclear disarmament and ecology is way above the norm. The level of culture is also abnormally high but not stuffy. The Davis Arts Centre is part-financed by the city and provides special tuition for talented children. However, the emphasis is on enabling and encouraging all the citizens of Davis to be creative whatever their talent. Concerts, exhibitions and shows given by the inhabitants are an everyday part of the Davis scene. The exceptionally low crime rate is thought to be partly a reflection of this communal interest in self-expression. Ecological awareness and creativity are considered good partners.

Richard St. George is a freelance environmental consultant, specializing in renewable energy and Green building.

Published in *Resurgence* No. 134, May/June 1989.

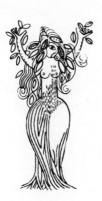